Sponsors

The 2nd Symposium on *Regulatory Autoantibodies Targeting G-Protein-Coupled Receptors* is kindly supported by

---

EUROIMMUN
a PerkinElmer company

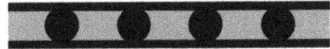

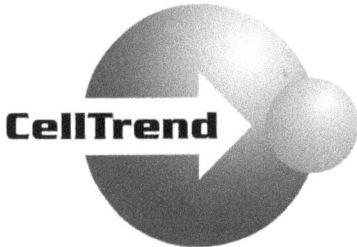

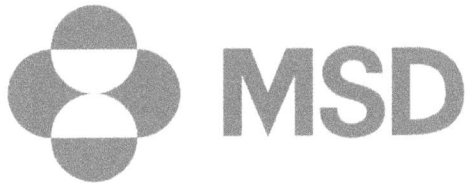

CellTrend

MSD

Bristol-Myers Squibb

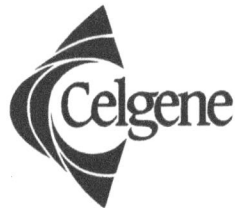

Celgene

SANOFI GENZYME

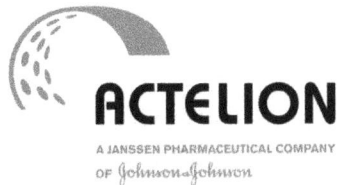

ACTELION
A JANSSEN PHARMACEUTICAL COMPANY
OF Johnson-Johnson

Sponsors cont´d

The 2nd Symposium on *Regulatory Autoantibodies Targeting G-Protein-Coupled Receptors* is kindly supported by

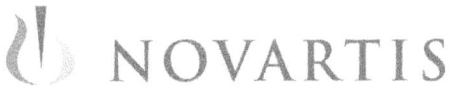

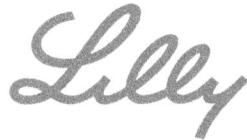

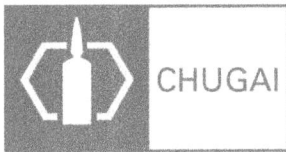

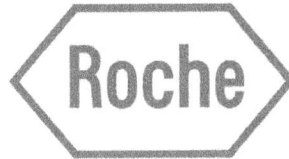

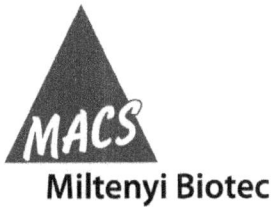

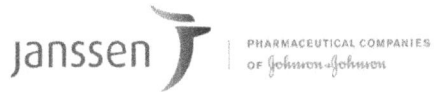

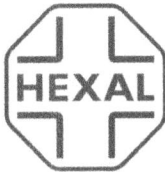

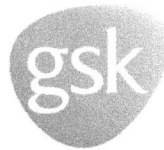

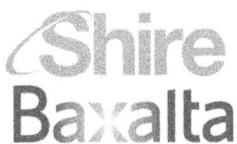

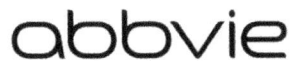

NOVARTIS

Lilly

CHUGAI

Roche

MACS
Miltenyi Biotec

Janssen
PHARMACEUTICAL COMPANIES
of Johnson-Johnson

HEXAL

gsk

Shire
Baxalta

abbvie

© 2018 Infinite Science Publishing
   University Press and
   Academic Printig

Imprint of Infinite Science GmbH,
MFC 1 | BioMedTec Wissenschaftscampus
Maria-Goeppert-Straße 1
23562 Lübeck

Cover Design: Infinite Science Publishing
Copy Editing: Department of Rheumatology, University of Lübeck and Infinite Science Publishing
Receptor illustration was generated by Anja Kerstein using PDB, OPM database and Jmol

Publisher: Infinite Science GmbH, Lübeck, www.infinite-science.de
Print: Norderstedt, Germany

ISBN Paperback: 978-3-945954-51-5

Bibliografische Information der Deutschen Nationalbibliothek:
Die Deutsche Nationalbibliothek verzeichnet diese Publikation in der Deutschen Nationalbibliografie; detaillierte bibliografische Daten sind im Internet über http://dnb.d-nb.de abrufbar.

Bibliographic information published by the Deutsche Nationalbibliothek
The Deutsche Nationalbibliothek lists this publication in the Deutsche Nationalbibliografie; detailed bibliographic data are available in the internet at http://dnb.d-nb.de.

Advances in RAB Research

2nd Symposium on
Regulatory Autoantibodies
Targeting G-Protein-Coupled
Receptors

Gabriela Riemekasten and
Anja Kerstein (Editors)
Department of Rheumatology
and Clinical Immunology
University of Lübeck

https://www.journals.infinite-science.de/rab

Infinite Science | Publishing

Recombinant Cell IFT (RC-IFT)

The fastest way from research to applied autoimmune diagnostics using indirect immunofluorescence

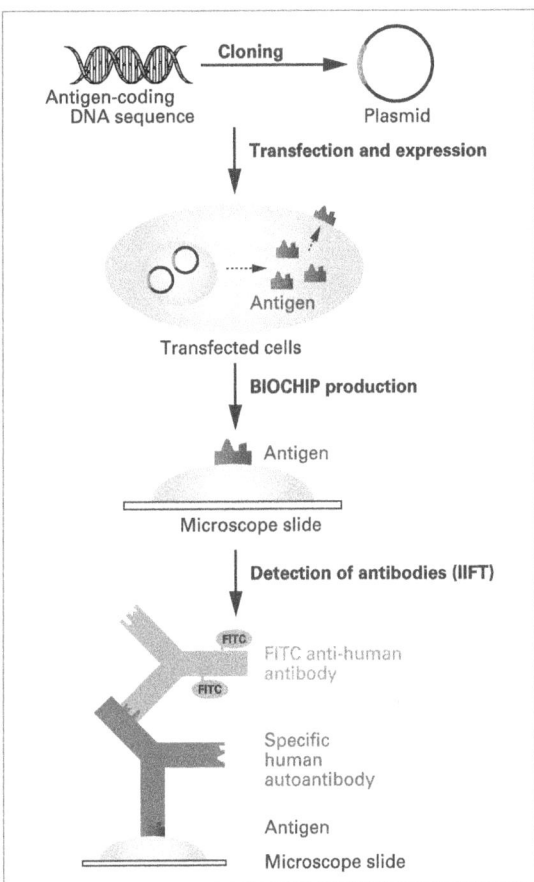

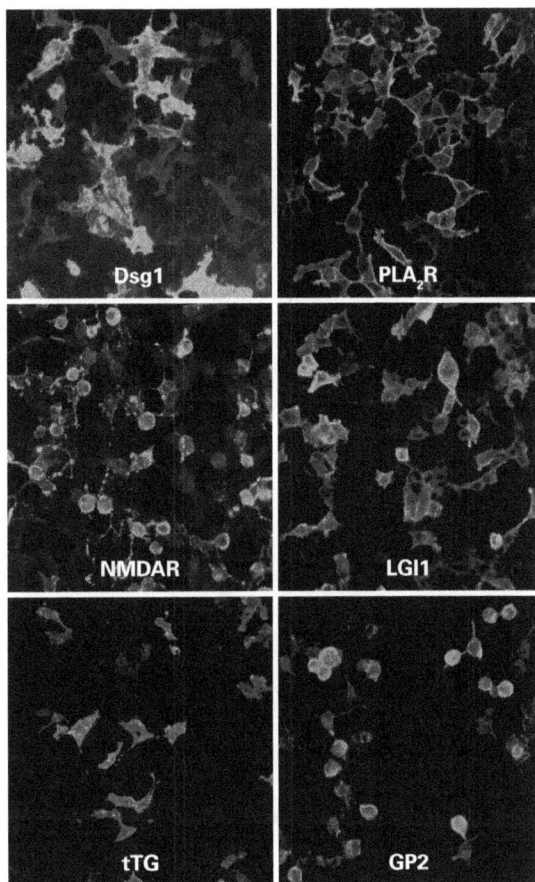

Cloning

Antigen-coding
DNA sequence

Plasmid

Transfection and expression

Antigen

Transfected cells

BIOCHIP production

Antigen

Microscope slide

Detection of antibodies (IIFT)

FITC anti-human
antibody

Specific
human
autoantibody

Antigen

Microscope slide

Dsg1 · PLA$_2$R · NMDAR · LGI1 · tTG · GP2

Detection of antibodies against

Skin antigens: desmoglein (Dsg) 1 and 3, BP230, collagen type VII, laminin 332**

Nephropathy-associated antigens: phospholipase-A$_2$ receptors (PLA$_2$R), thrombospondin type-1 domain-containing protein 7A (THSD7A)

Neural antigens: glutamate receptors type NMDA, type AMPA, VGKC (LGI1, CASPR2), GABA$_B$ receptors, DPPX, glycine receptors**, aquaporin-4, MOG, Tr (DNER), ITPR1*, CARP*, Yo/CDR2*, ZIC4, IgLON5, mGluR5*, flotillin1/2*

Further antigens: pancreas antigens rPAg1 (CUZD1) and rPAg2 (GP2), glutamic acid decarboxylase (GAD65), SLA/LP, TIF1-gamma, tissue transglutaminase (tTG)**

*Currently not available as IVD in the EU   **In development

CellTrend

ELISA

for Detection
of Antibodies
against:

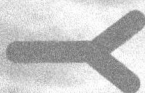

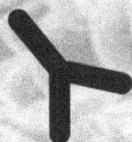

GPCRs
(e.g. AT1R)

TKR
(e.g. VEGF-R1)

(e.g. VEGF-A)

CellTrend GmbH
Im Biotechnologiepark 3 • TGZ II • 14943 Luckenwalde
Tel: + (0) 33 71/ 61 99 600 • www.celltrend.de

Ein forschendes BioPharma-Unternehmen.

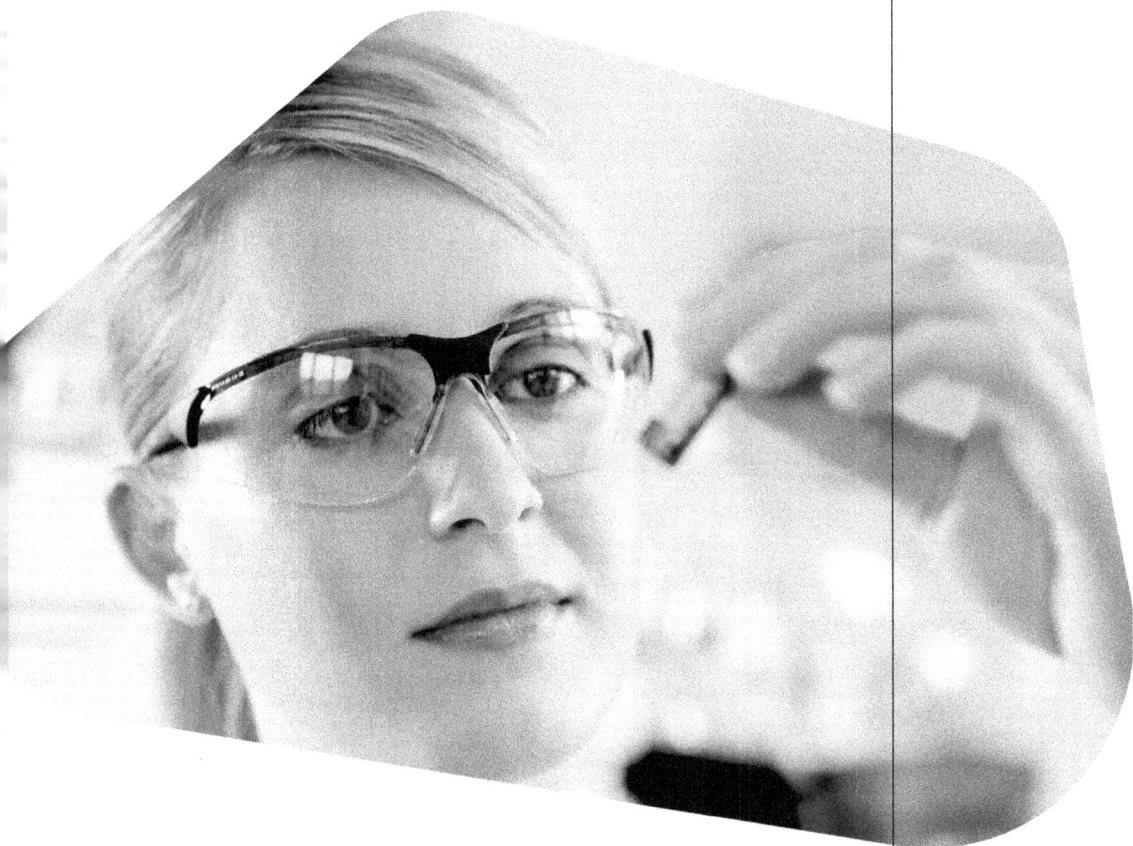

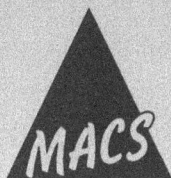

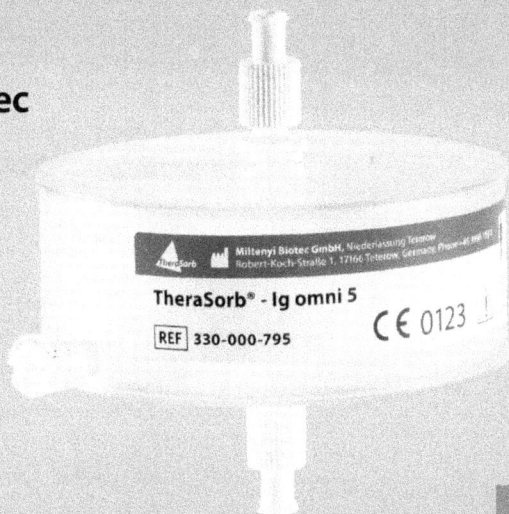

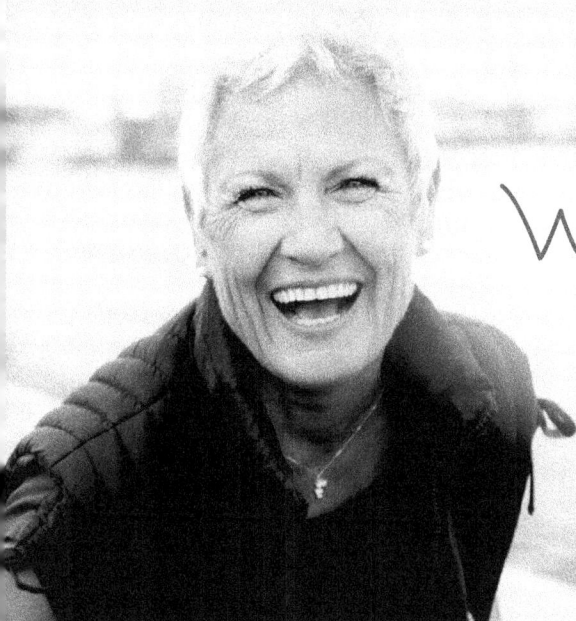

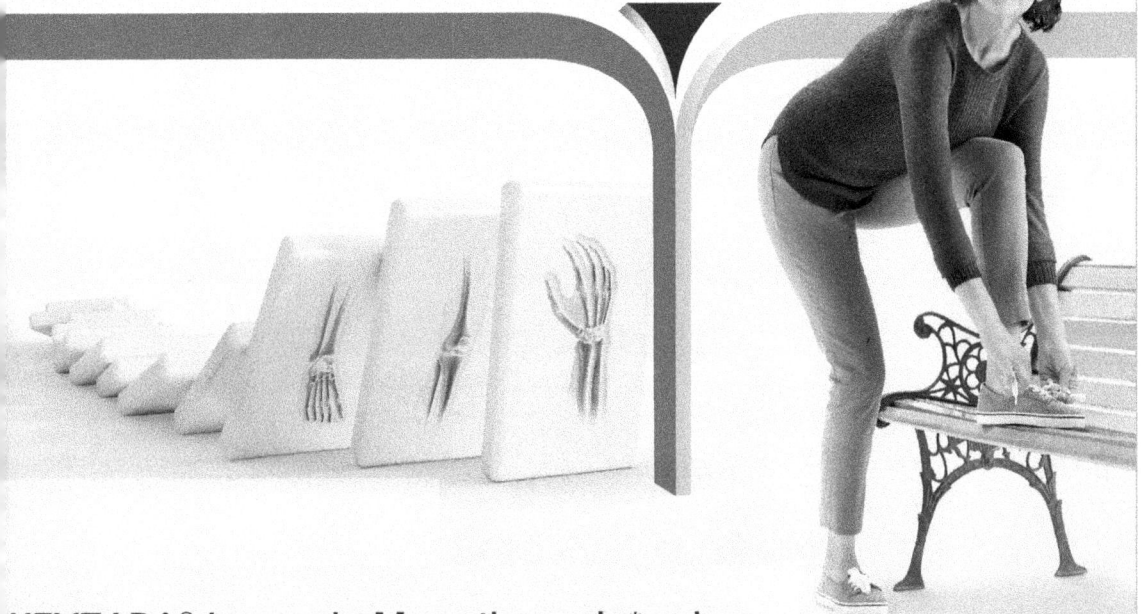

CHUGAI

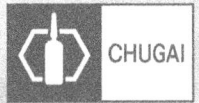

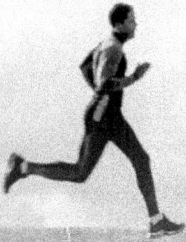

UNSER WEG ZU INNOVATION:
Talent und Technologie

Für Patienten in der Hämophilie,
Rheumatologie und Onkologie.

中外製薬
INNOVATION BEYOND IMAGINATION

Program Committee

Prof. Dr. Gabriela Riemekasten
Director, Department of Rheumatology
and Clinical Immunology
Universitätsklinikum Schleswig-Holstein
Universität zu Lübeck

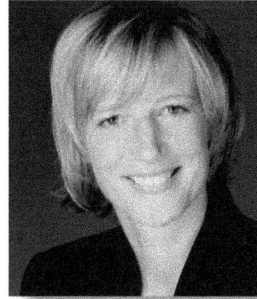

Prof. Dr. Yehuda Shoenfeld
Head of the Center of Autoimmunity at Sheba
Head The Mosaic of Autoimmunity Project of
Saint Petersburg University
Tel Ha Shomer Hospital
Tel Aviv University, Isreal

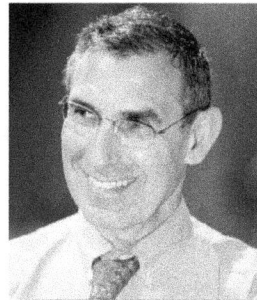

Prof. Dr. Duska Dragun
Head of the Nephrology Research Laboratory
at the Charité Campus Virchow-Klinikum
Berlin

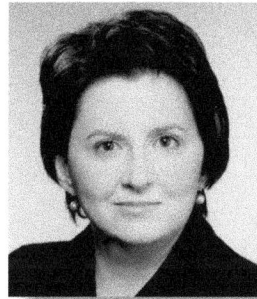

Prof. Dr. Fritz Boege
Director, Central Institute for Clinical Chemistry
and Laboratory Diagnostics
Universitätsklinikum Düsseldorf

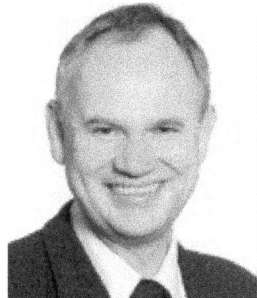

Preface

Greeting from the Symposium Chair

Dear Sir or Madam, Dear Colleagues,

It is a great pleasure to announce our second symposium on functional or regulatory autoantibodies targeting G-protein-coupled receptors (GPCRs) in Lübeck.

GPCRs are involved in a variety of physiological and pathophysiological processes. So far, much effort has been made on anti-GPCR drug discovery with a focus on the development of small molecules for the treatment of cancer, infection, metabolic disorders or inflammatory diseases.

Recently, functional autoantibodies against GPCRs were identified in healthy donors and were found to be dysregulated in various diseases. They are associated with pathogenesis, uncovering a potential new field of therapeutic intervention.

Thus, the aim of this symposium is to combine the current knowledge about the role of anti-GPCR ab in different pathologies, their mode of action and state-of-the-art research techniques to identify common fundamental pathways that can be transferred to other disease entities with similar manifestations.

I cordially invite you to participate in this inspiring symposium with outstanding speakers from the field of GPCR research and constructive discussions as well as poster sessions.

I look forward to welcome you to the beautiful Hanseatic City of Lübeck and encourage you and your colleagues to contribute to this exciting meeting.

Prof. Dr. Gabriela Riemekasten
Director, Department of Rheumatology and Clinical Immunology
University of Lübeck, Germany

Table of Contents

Monoclonal anti-AT1R ab from a SSc mouse model: evaluation of their functions

Frank Petersen   1809010

Transfer of PBMC from SSc patients to immunodeficient mice leads to the production of autoantibodies against AT1R and ETAR

Xiaoyang Yue, Yaqing Shu, Junie Tchudjin Magatsin, Xiaoqing Wang, Junping Yin Marjan Ahmadi, Harald Heidecke, Brigitte Kasper, Xinhua Yu, Frank Petersen, Gabriela Riemekasten   1809011

Section 4: Signaling of anti -GPCR ab: can we identify novel targets?

Signaling and GPCR biology using cell models

Philippe Aurélie   1809012

Lessons from dermatology: Anti-Dsg1/3 und anti-BP180-induced signaling

Ralf Ludwig   1809013

Role of antibodies against PAR-1 and PAR-2 in cancer in the kidney transplant recipients

R. Catara, R. Carroll, L. Chen, Q. Li, I. Schramm, M. Simon, O. Wischnewski, A. Kusch, A. Philippe, D. Dragun   1809014

Sialylated autoantigen-reactive IgG antibodies attenuate disease development in mouse models of lupus nephritis and rheumatoid arthritis

Yannic C. Bartsch, Johann Rahmöller, Alexei Leliavski, Gina-Maria Lilienthal, Janina Petry, Marc Ehlers   1809015

Autoantibodies targeting complement receptors 3a and 5a are decreased in ANCA-associated vasculitis

Sebastian Klapa, Andreas Koch, Anja Kerstein, Christian Karsten, Harald Heidecke, Markus Huber-Lang, Peter Lamprecht, Gabriela Riemekasten, Antje Müller   1809016

Impact of regulatory (auto-)antibodies against G-protein-coupled receptors on blood pressure in women ten years after early-onset preeclampsia

Anna Birukov, Hella Muijsers, Harald Heidecke, Nadine Haase, Kristin Kräker, Dominik N. Müller, Florian Herse, Angela Maas, Ralf Dechend   1809017

Section 5: Anti -GPCR ab as marker for diseases and therapeutic responses

Antibodies against complement receptors: impact on pathophysiology

Christian Karsten   1809018

Anti-GPCR antibodies in atherosclerosis

Zouhair Aherrahrou, Laurence Johanson, Jeanette Erdmann,
Gabriela Riemekasten   1809019

Immunoadsorption in Vascular Dementia - a novel approach to Alzheimer´s
Disease?

Hans Jörgen Grabe   1809020

First results of the prospective ETiCS-study: acute (microbial-associated)
inflammation rather than (infarction-associated) myocardial ischemia triggers
the development of cardiac GPCR autoantibodies

Valérie Boivin-Jahns, Chistina Zechmeister, Claudia Schuetz, Niklas Beyersdorf,
Stefan Stoerk, Roland Jahns   1809021

Section 6: How to target effects of functional antibodies

Immunoadsorption to remove ß adrenergic and M acetylcholine receptor
antibodies in Chronic Fatigue Syndrome (CFS/ME)

Carmen Scheibenbogen, Markus Tölle, Antonia Berz, Helma Freitag, Franziska
Sotzny, Wolfram Doehner, Nadja Scherbakov, Sandra Bauer, Michaela
Antelmann, Harald Heidecke, Patricia Grabowski   1809022

The aptamer BC 007 completely neutralizes agonistic autoantibodies directed
against β1-adrenoceptors: Results of a phase 1 trial

Niels-Peter Becker, Johannes Mueller, Annekathrin Haberland, Katrin Wenzel,
Gerd Wallukat, Peter Goettel, Sarah Schulze- Rothe, Ingolf Schimke,
Georg Golor, Matthias Grossmann, Angela Sinn, Martina Steiper, Tuba Yilmaz,
Anne Wallukat, Hanna Davideit, Susanne Becker   1809023

Agonistic antibody diseases = Autoimmune diseases? From bench to bedside

Rudolf Kunze   1809024

Autoantibodies in serum of systemic scleroderma patients: peptide-based
epitope mapping indicates increased binding to cytoplasmic domains of CXCR3

Andreas Recke, Ann-Katrin Regensburger, Florian Weigold, Antje Müller, Harald
Heidecke, Gabriele Marschner, Christoph M. Hammers, Ralf J. Ludwig, Gabriela
Riemekastenb   1809025

Detection and functional characterization of angiotensin receptor Type 1
autoantibodies: establishment and clinical translation

Valérie Boivin-Jahns, Chistina Zechmeister, Claudia Schuetz, Martin J. Lohse,
Roland Jahns, Xinhua Yu, Frank Petersen, Stefanie Hahner, Martin Fassnacht   1809026

Section 7: Posters

Autoantibodies targeting G-protein-coupled receptors in RA and SLE	P01
Xiaoyang Xiaoyang, Qiaoniang Huang, Fengyuan Deng, Fengyuan Deng, Juan Chen, Harald Heidecke, Gabriela Riemekasten, Frank Petersen, Xinhua Yu	1809027
Identification and characterization of cytomegalovirus-specific CD8+ T cells in systemic sclerosis	P02
Gesa Balsen, Antje Müller, Silke Pitann, Kerstin Mosenthin, Stoyan Dimitrov, Gabriela Riemekasten, Tanja Lange	1809028
Organotropism of anti-CXCR3/4- and anti-ETAR/-AT1Rmediated leukocyte migration in inflammatory and autoimmune disease	P03
Laurence Johansona, Antje Müller, Zouhair Aherrahrou, Jennifer Hundt, Anja Kerstein, Gabriele Marschner, Silke Pitann, Sara Comdühr, Gesche Weppner, Harald Heidecke, Peter Lamprecht , Christiane Herden, Gabriela Riekemasten	1809029
Autoantibodies targeting muscarinic acetylcholine receptors: implications on fatigue in systemic sclerosis	P04
Sabine Sommerlatte, Hannah Bittern, Silke Pitann, Gabriele Marschner, Antje Müller, Otavio Cabral-Marques, Harald Heidecke, Tanja Lange, Gabriela Riemekasten	1809030
Role of anti-alpha-adrenoceptor autoantibodies and leukocytic alpha-adrenoceptors in primary Raynaud's phenomenon	P05
Catharina Frahm, Anja Kerstein, Silke Pitann, Sara Comdühr, Harald Heidecke, Antje Müller, Tanja Lange, Gabriela Riemekasten	1809031
Inflamed tissue contributes to the emergence of autoreactivity in granulomatosis with polyangiitis	P06
Gesche Weppner, Olena Ohlei, Christoph M. Hammers, Konstanze Holl-Ulrich, Jan Voswinkel, Julia Bischof, Katrin Hasselbacher, Gabriela Riemekasten, Peter Lamprecht, Saleh Ibrahim, Christof Iking-Konert, Andreas Recke, Antje Müller	1809032
New insights into the diagnostics of autoantibodies against G-protein coupled receptors – pitfalls in the autoantibody detection	P07
Annekathrin Haberland, Johannes Müller, Gerd Wallukat, Katrin Wenzel	1809033
Network-based analysis reveals signatures of IgG autoantibodies targeting G protein-coupled receptors in health and disease	P08
Otavio Cabral-Marques, Alexandre Marques, Lasse Melvær Giil, Roberta de Vito, Barbara Elizabeth Engelhardt, Jalid Sehouli, Harald Heidecke, Gabriela Riemekasten	1809002
β1-adrenergic receptor autoantibody levels are higher in patients with Graves' hyperthyroidism than in matched healthy controls and decrease after antithyroid treatment	P09
Anna Lundgren, Karin Tammelin, Mats Holmberg, Helena Filipsson Nyström	1809005

Patterns of 31 new autoantibodies against G-protein-coupled receptors and growth factors	P10
H. Bittern, A. Carvalho-Marques, C. Fouodo, I. König, S. Schinke, O. Cabral-Marques, H. Heidecke, G. Riemekasten	1809006
Transfer of PBMC from SSc patients to immunodeficient mice leads to the production of autoantibodies against AT1R and ETAR	P11
Xiaoyang Yue, Yaqing Shu, Junie Tchudjin Magatsin, Xiaoqing Wang, Junping Yin Marjan Ahmadi, Harald Heidecke, Brigitte Kasper, Xinhua Yu, Frank Petersen, Gabriela Riemekasten	1809011
Sialylated autoantigen-reactive IgG antibodies attenuate disease development in mouse models of lupus nephritis and rheumatoid arthritis	P12
Yannic C. Bartsch, Johann Rahmöller, Alexei Leliavski, Gina-Maria Lilienthal, Janina Petry, Marc Ehlers	1809015
Autoantibodies targeting complement receptors 3a and 5a are decreased in ANCA-associated vasculitis	P13
Sebastian Klapa, Andreas Koch, Anja Kerstein, Christian Karsten, Harald Heidecke, Markus Huber-Lang, Peter Lamprecht, Gabriela Riemekasten, Antje Müller	1809016
Impact of regulatory (auto-)antibodies against G-protein-coupled receptors on blood pressure in women ten years after early-onset preeclampsia	P14
Anna Birukov, Hella Muijsers, Harald Heidecke, Nadine Haase, Kristin Kräker, Dominik N. Müller, Florian Herse, Angela Maas, Ralf Dechend	1809017
Autoantibodies in serum of systemic scleroderma patients: peptide-based epitope mapping indicates increased binding to cytoplasmic domains of CXCR3	P15
Andreas Recke, Ann-Katrin Regensburger, Florian Weigold, Antje Müller, Harald Heidecke, Gabriele Marschner, Christoph M. Hammers, Ralf J. Ludwig, Gabriela Riemekastenb	1809025
Detection and functional characterization of angiotensin receptor Type 1 autoantibodies: establishment and clinical translation	P16
Valérie Boivin-Jahns, Chistina Zechmeister, Claudia Schuetz, Martin J. Lohse, Roland Jahns, Xinhua Yu, Frank Petersen, Stefanie Hahner, Martin Fassnacht	1809026

Section 1
Opening Lectures

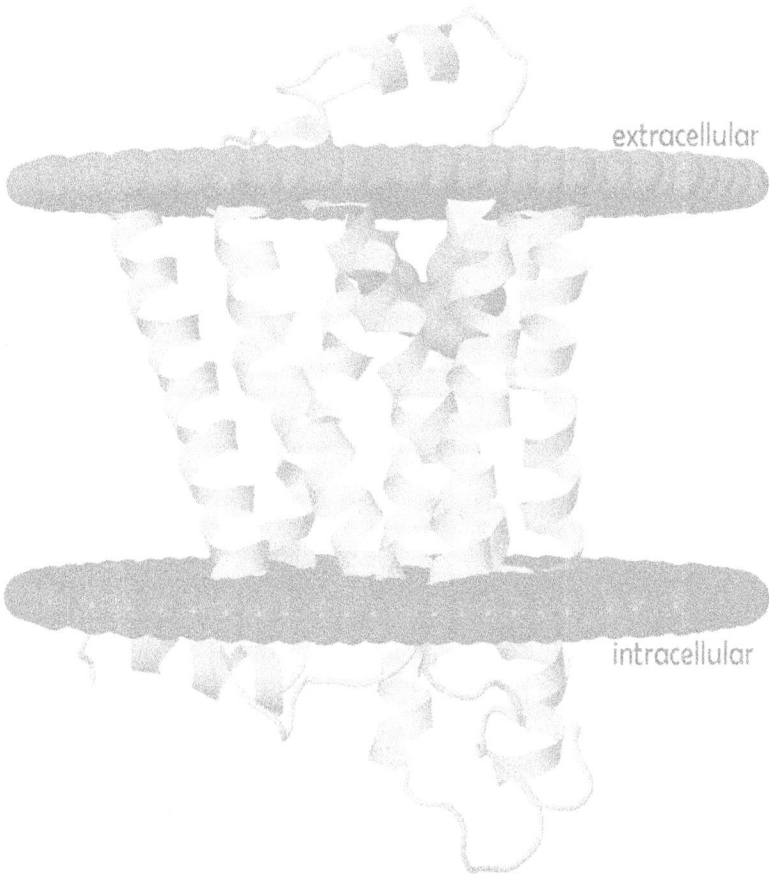

extracellular

intracellular

The mosaic of autoimmunity: Why we develop autoimmune diseases. The microbiome and metabolism

Yehuda Shoenfeld

Zabludowicz Center for Autoimmune Diseases, Sheba Medical Center, Tel Aviv University, Israel
Past incumbent of the Laura Schwartz Kipp Chair for Research of Autoimmune Diseases. Sackler
Faculty of Medicine, Tel Aviv University, Israel
Corresponding author, email: shoenfel@post.tau.ac.il

Background: Autoimmune diseases are conditions in which the immune system damages normal components of the individual. Initially it was thought that autoimmune disease was the inevitable outcome of the presence of clones of lymphocytes with receptors that recognize self-antigens. Thus tolerance to self, the state of non-autoimmunity, was due to the absence of self-recognizing lymphocytes, the 'forbidden' culprits of autoimmune disease. Autoimmune diseases were found to be multifactorial in their etiology. For practical reasons these factors are classified into four categories:

Genetic, which entail the MHC class I, II, and III. A case in point will be the haplotypes of HLA-DRB1 which are prevalent in many classical diseases.

Immune deficiencies: C1q C2, C4 and IgA deficiencies are among the most common defects associated with diverse autoimmune conditions.

Hormonal state, most autoimmune diseases are detected in females at the child bearing ages. The role of estrogens will be delineated. In addition, other hormones play a role i.e. prolactin.

Environmental causes: Those are the most important as a trigger factors determining the time and type of disease. They entail infectious agents, chemicals, adjuvants, drugs and even vaccines. We will discuss smoking, different types of food (i.e. salt, coffee, chocolate, spicy food, etc.) and their effect on the microbiome.

The type of disease in an individual, in an autoimmune prone family, will be determined by the specific combination of the different factors mentioned above. A special emphasis will be put on the component of parasites.

DOI: 10.18416/RAB.2018.1809001   Advances in RAB Research • Article ID: 1809001

Infinite Science
Publishing

References:

1) Shoenfeld Y, et al. The mosaic of autoimmunity. IAMJ 2008; 10; pp. 3-7; 8-12; 13-19.

2) Yaxiong Deng, Xin Huang, Haijing Wu, Ming Zhao, Qianjin Lu, Eitan Israeli, Shani Dahan, Miri Blank, Yehuda Shoenfeld. Some like it hot: The emerging role of spicy food (capsaicin) in 3 autoimmune diseases. Autoimmunity Reviews 2016; 15(5): 451-456.

3) Carlo Perricone, Mathilde Versini, Dana Ben-Ami, Smadar Gertel, Abdulla Watad, Michael J. Segel, Fulvia Ceccarelli, Fabrizio Conti, Luca Cantarini, Dimitrios P. Bogdanos, Alessandro Antonelli, Howard Amital, Guido Valesini, Yehuda Shoenfeld. Smoke and autoimmunity: The fire behind the disease. Autoimmunity Reviews 2016; 15: 354–374.

4) Katchan V, David P, Shoenfeld Y. Cannabinoids and autoimmune diseases: A systematic review. Autoimmunity Reviews 2016; 15: 513–528.

Network-based analysis reveals signatures of IgG autoantibodies targeting G protein-coupled receptors in health and disease

Otavio Cabral-Marques[a], Alexandre Marques[a], Lasse Melvær Giil[b], Roberta de Vito[c], Barbara Elizabeth Engelhardt[c], Jalid Sehouli[d], Harald Heidecke[e], Gabriela Riemekasten[a,*]

[a] Department of Rheumatology and Clinical Immunology, University of Lübeck, Lübeck, Germany
[b] Deaconess Hospital, University of Bergen, Bergen, Norway
[c] Department of Computer Science, Princeton University, Princeton, NJ, USA
[d] Department of Gynecology, Charité University Hospital, Berlin and Tumor Bank Ovarian Cancer Network (TOC), Berlin, Germany
[e] CellTrend GmbH, Luckenwalde, Brandenburg, Germany
[*] Corresponding author, email: Gabriela.Riemekasten@uksh.de

Background: Functional antibodies (ab) against G protein-coupled receptors (GPCR) were found in various diseases and partially in healthy individuals. Their role in physiology and in pathophysiology remains to be identified.

Methods: Sera from 952 patients with different rheumatic diseases were analyzed for the presence of ten different anti-GPCR ab by ELISAs. For deeper ab phenotyping, ab levels against 30 different autoantigens including GPCR, growth factors, and growth factor receptors were studied in sera from 491 healthy controls (HC), 84 patients with systemic sclerosis, 91 with Alzheimer's disease, and 207 with ovarian cancer by ELISAs. Spearman's rank correlation coefficients, hierarchical cluster analyses, network mapping and target interactions using STRING and gene ontology (GO) analyses were performed as well as transwell migration assays.

Results: Specific signatures were identified in different autoimmune diseases and in HC. Ab correlations and clusters of correlations were identified in HC, which were specifically affected by age, sex, and autoimmune and non-autoimmune diseases. Network mapping and GO analysis of ab targets displayed multiple associations and a central role of the endothelin receptor type-A (ETAR) in cell migration and chemoattraction. Indeed, the ab were chemoattractive for immune cells, which could be ameliorated by ETAR blockers.

Conclusions: Our data indicate a functional ab network, which is affected by age, sex, and diseases. The network could affect receptor functions and could guide immune cells or their targets via chemoattraction to organs.

DOI: 10.18416/RAB.2018.1809002   Advances in RAB Research • Article ID: 1809002

Section 2

Anti-GPCR ab: advantages, pitfalls and problems in the diagnosis

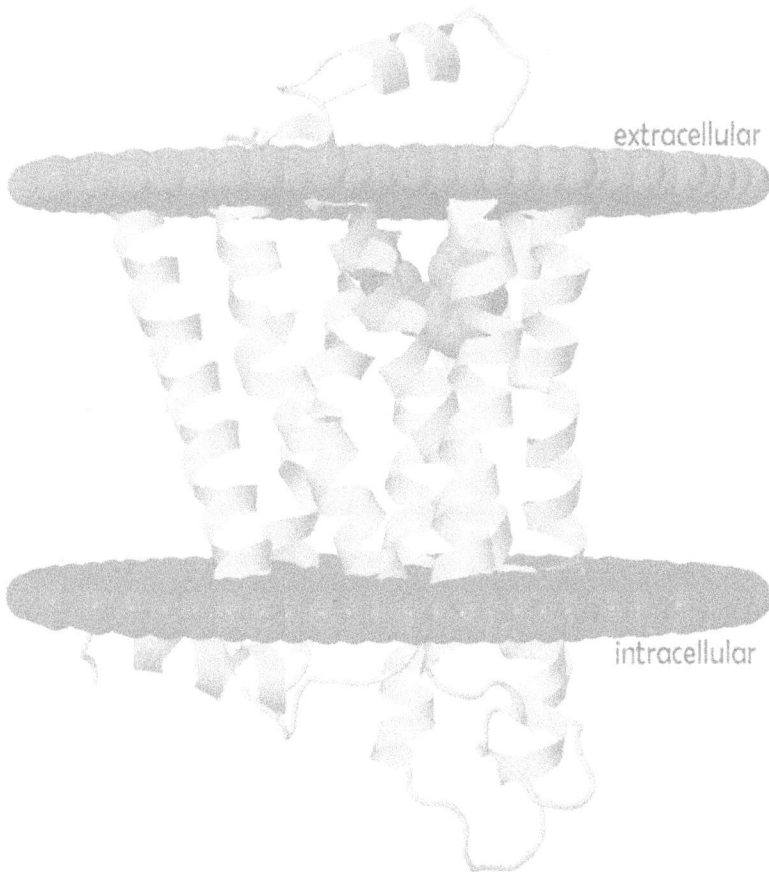

To smell the SLE-CNS involvement

Yehuda Shoenfeld

Zabludowicz Center for Autoimmune Diseases, Sheba Medical Center, Tel Aviv University, Israel
Past incumbent of the Laura Schwartz Kipp Chair for Research of Autoimmune Diseases. Sackler
Faculty of Medicine, Tel Aviv University, Israel
Corresponding author, email: shoenfel@post.tau.ac.il

Central Nervous System involvement in Systemic Lupus Erythematosus (**CNS-SLE**) is very common and ranges between 20% – 70% of the patients. The CNS involvement is listed in the ARA criteria for SLE diagnosis.

CNS-SLE is associated with more than 20 different autoantibodies (1). Yet, remarkable among them are the **anti-P-ribosomal antibodies** (anti-PR) (2). These autoantibodies directed mainly against the carboxy 22 amino acids of the PO, P1 P2 ribosomal phosphoproteins. They are capable of penetrating lived cells and inducing apoptotic changes as well as leading to inhibition of specific cytokine secretion (3-5). The titer of the autoantibodies correlates with disease activity, kidney involvement and hepatitis (6-8).

Anti-PR were first reported to associate and correlate with CNS-SLE and especially psychosis in 1987(9). Subsequent analyses could only partially repeat Bonfa's conclusions (2-3). The contradictory results may stem from technical discrepancies (2-3), multiplicity of autoantibodies causing CNS-SLE (1,10), and differences in the time of drawing the blood in relation to the time when the patient had the CNS involvement.

We employed affinity purified anti-PR on a PR column and injected them directly into the brain ventricles of Balb/c mice. Irrelevant Igs were employed as controls. The analyses entailed a variety of neurological tests known to evaluate cognitive impairment, anxiety states, depressive conditions and motor competence of the mice.

Mice injected with anti-PR clearly expressed **depressive behavior**, characterized mainly by floating pattern rather than swimming in an enforced swimming tests. These floating pattern could be reversed by a specific therapy with monoclonal anti-idiotypic antibody to anti-PR (11), by IVIG as well as Fluoxetine (Prozac) an anti-depression drug. No response was achieved with anti-psychotic drug. The control mice were not affected in their behavior following the injection of the irrelevant Ig (12).

The human purified anti-P-R, were shown to bind to CNS structures consisting with the **smell apparatus** (i.e. amygdale, hypocampus and other parts of the limbic systems).

Smell defects characterize bulbectomized (cutting the olfactory nerves) depressive mice (13), as well as depressive women (14). Such depression can be overcome by exposing mice and humans to citrus fragrance (15).

Our studies show for the first time the active induction of a psychiatric condition (i.e. depression) with a specific autoantibody, i.e. **anti-PR** (16). Furthermore, the results allude to a novel mechanism to explain the induction of CNS-SLE depression (i.e. involvement of the smell apparatus).

These data may pave the road to a novel approach to depression in CNS-SLE and its therapy as well as in other CNS conditions (12,17,18-21).

References:

1) Gisele Zandman-Goddard, Joab Chapman, Yehuda Shoenfeld.Explosion of autoantibodies involved in neuropsychiatric. SLE and antiphospholipid syndrome. (Submitted to Seminars in Arthritis and Rheumatism, 2006).

2) Eber T, Chapman J, Shoenfeld Y. Anti-ribosimal P-protein and its role in psychiatric manifestations of systemic lupus erythematosus: myth or reality? Lupus 1005; 14: 571-5.

3) Gerli R, Caponi L. Anti-ribosomal P protein antibodies. Autoimmunity 2005; 38: 85-92.

4) Sun KJ, et al. Monoclonal ribosomal P autoantibody inhibits the expression and release of IL-12, TNF-alpha and iNOS in activated RAW macrophage cell line. J Autoimmun 2005; 24: 135-43.

5) Nagai T, Arinuma Y, Yanagida T, Yamamoto K, Hirohata S. Anti-ribosomal P protein antibody in human systemic lupus erythematosus up-regulates the expression of proinflammatory cytokines by human peripheral blood monoclytes. Arthritis Rheum 2005; 52: 847-55.

6) Karassa FB, et al. Accuracy of anti-ribosomal P protein antibody testing for the diagnosis of neuropsychiatric systemic lupus erythematosus: and international meta-analysis. Arthritis Rheum 2006; 54: 312-24.

7) do Nascimento AP, Viana Vdos S, Testagrossa Lde A, Leon EP, Borda EF, Barros Rt, Bonfa E. Antibodies to ribosomal P proteins: a potential serologic marker for lupus membranous glomerulonephritis. Arthritis Rheum 2006; 54: 1568-72.

8) Takeda I, et al. Anti-ribosimal p antibodies are associated with nephritis, vascular thrombosis and lymphocytopenia in patients with systemic lupus erythematosus. Fukushima J Med Sci 2005; 51: 11-8.

9) Bonfa E, Golombek SJ, Kaufman LD, Skelly S, Weissbach H, Brot N, Elkon KB. Association between lupus psychosis and anti-ribosomal P protein antibodies. New Engl J Med 1987; 317: 265-71.

10) Shovman O, Gilburd B, Barzilai O, Shinar E, Larida B, Zandman-Goddard G, Binder SR, Shoenfeld Y. Evaluation of the BioPlex 2200 ANA screen: analysis of 510 healthy subjects: incidence of natural/predictive autoantibodies. Ann NY Acad Sci 2005; 1050: 380-8.

11) Zhang W, Reichlin M. Production and characterization of a human monoclonal anti-idiotype to anti-ribosomal P antibodies. Clin Immunol 2005; 114: 130-6.

12) Katzav A, Solodeev I, Brodsky O, Chapman J, Pick CG, Blank M, Zhang W, Reichlin M, Shoenfeld Y. Induction of autoimmune depression in mice by anti-ribosomal P antibodies via the limbic system. Arth & Rheum 56: 938-948, 2007.

13) Zueger M, Urani A, Chourbaji S, Zacher C, Roche M, Harkin A, Gass P. Olfactory bulbectomy in mice induces alterations in exploratory behavior. Neurosci Lett. 2005; 374: 142-6.

14) Satoh S, Morita N, Matsuzaki I, Konishi T, Nakano T, Minoshita S, Arizono H, Saito S, Avabe AS. Relationship between odor perception aqnd depression in the Japanese elderly. Psychiatry Clin Neurosci 1996; 50: 2781-5.

15) Komori T, Fujiwara R, Tanida M, Nomura J, Yokoyama MM. Effects of citrus fragrance on immune function and depressive states. Meuroimmunomodulation 1995; 2: 174-180.

16) Yoshio T, et al. Antiribosomal P protein antibodies in cerebrospinal fluid are associated with neuropsychiatric systemic lupus erythematosus. J Rheumatol 2005; 32: 334-9.

17) Zivadinov R, Zorzon M, Monti Bragadin L, Pagliarto G, Cazzato G. Olfactory loss in multiple sclerosis. Meurol Scio, 1999; 168: 127-30.

18) Shoenfeld Y. To smell autoimmunity: Anti-P-Ribosomal autoantibodies, depression, and the olfactory system. J Autoimmunity 28: 165-169, 2007.

19) Secundo L, Snitz K, Weissler K, Pinchover L, Shoenfeld Y, Loewenthal R, Agmon-Levin N, Frumin I, Bar-Zvi D, Shushan S, Sobel N. Individual olfactory perception reveals meaningful nonolfactory genetic information. Proc Natl Acad Sci USA 2015; 14: 112: 8750-5.

20). Rattazzi L, Cariboni A, Poojara R, Shoenfeld Y, D'Acquisto F. Impaired sense of smell and altered olfactory system in RAG-1 -/- immunodeficient mice. Frontiers in Nuroscience 2015; volume 9, Article 318.

21) Shamriz O, Shoenfeld Y. Olfactory dysfunction and autoimmunity: pathogenesis and new insights. Clin Exp Rheumatol 2017; 35: 1037-1042.

Lessons From Anti-TSH-Receptor Autoantibodies: Challenges And Pitfalls In Diagnostics

Paul J Banga[a], Simon D. Lytton[b,*]

[a] *King's College London Faculty of Life Sciences & Medicine Denmark Hill Campus London, SE5 9PJ UK*
[b] *SeraDiaLogistics, Munich. Germany*
[*] *Corresponding author, email: simon.lytton@t-online.de*

Objective: Autoantibodies to the thyrotropin hormone receptor (TSH-R) directly mediate Graves' disease (GD) and orbital manifestations of Graves' orbitopathy (GO). To explore their heterogeneous function, TSH-R autoantibody binding in immunoassays (TRAb) versus their functional activity; stimulators of cAMP in bioassay (TSIs or TSAbs) or inhibitors of the thyrotropic hormone (TSH) binding to TSH-R, detected by decreased cAMP in bioassay (TBAbs), is assessed.

Methods: TRAb measurements by automated electrochemical luminescence immunoassays (ECLIA) and stimulating and blocking activity on Chinese hamster ovary cell (CHO) Mc4 bioassays (Thyretain ®, Quidel). The activity of patient immunoglobulins on ECLIA; M22 Mab competition (cobas elecsys, Roche) or TSH-R bridge assay (Immulite,Siemens) versus Mc4 TSI bioassay were correlated with GO clinical activity by meta-analysis of complete Pubmed-published data sets (n=5).

Results: The automated ECLIA show less sensitivity than cell-based bioassay for detection of TRAbs (Fig 1A and 1B) and do not distinguish between stimulator MAbs; M22 and KSAb (Fig 1A and 1B) versus the blocker MAb K1-70 (Fig 1C). In contrast, Mc4 TSAb bioassay of K1-70 detected null stimulatory activity (Fig 1C), in contrast to strong cAMP inhibition in Mc4 TBAb blocker reporter bioassay (Fig 1D). Diagnostic performances of Mc4 TSAb bioassay and automated TRAb ECLIA in untreated GD show high sensitivities 97% (95-100) and specificities 98% (96-100%). Meta-analysis of GD and/or GO undergoing treatment reveal lower percent positive on Mc4 TSI Bioassay (56%, range 13-87%) than ECLIA TRAb immunoassays (98.5%, range 98-99%; OR=2.76, p=0.09). The Forest plot total random effects of correlation coefficients of autoantibody activity with GO clinical activity were greater on Mc4 bioassay (r=0.4, I2 =92% (95% CI 89-95), p<0.0.001) versus TRAb immunoassay (r=0.2, I2 =39% (95% CI 0-70%), p=0.0.8).

Conclusion: Diagnostic distinction of TSAbs and TBAbs is of paramount clinical importance. Cell-based bioassays are the only method to distinguish between TSAbs and TBAbs. To avoid the pitfall of incorrect reporting on automated TRAb binding assays, TSI or TSAb is strongly recommended for results of bioassays; whereas the results of automated ECLIA should be reported as TRAbs (of undetermined functional significance).

DOI: 10.18416/RAB.2018.1809004   Advances in RAB Research • Article ID: 1809004

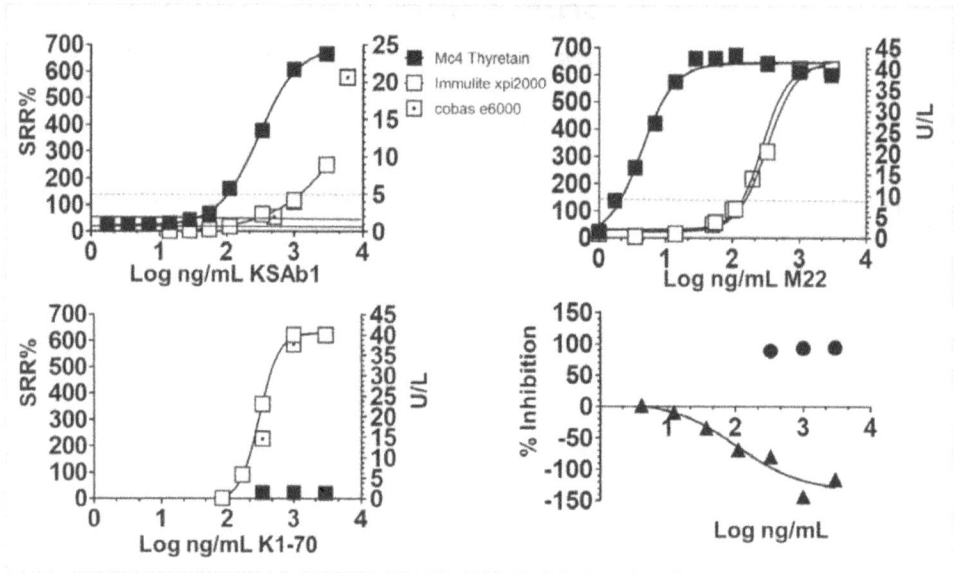

Figure 1. *Analytical sensitivity of the TSH-R bioassays versus binding immunoassays. Titration of the concentrations of anti-TSH-R monoclonal autoantibodies A) mouse stimulatory KSAb1 (22,40) B) human stimulatory M22 (RSR Ltd Cardiff UK, Cat Nr M22/FD/0.0*

Reference: Frontiers in Bioscience, Landmark, 23, 2028-2043, 2018.

β1-adrenergic receptor autoantibody levels are higher in patients with Graves' hyperthyroidism than in matched healthy controls and decrease after anti-thyroid treatment

Anna Lundgren[a,*], Karin Tammelin[b], Mats Holmberg[c], Helena Filipsson Nyström[d]

[a] *Clinical Immunology and Transfusion Medicine, Sahlgrenska University Hospital, Gothenburg, Sweden*
[b] *Department of Medicine, Sahlgrenska University Hospital/Östra, Gothenburg, Sweden*
[c] *Institute of Medicine, Sahlgrenska Academy, University of Gothenburg, Gothenburg, Sweden and ANOVA, Karolinska University Hospital, Stockholm, Sweden*
[d] *Department of Endocrinology, Sahlgrenska University Hospital, Gothenburg, Sweden*
[*] *Corresponding author, email: anna.e.lundgren@vgregion.se*

Background: Graves' disease (GD) is driven by autoantibodies targeting the thyroid-stimulating hormone receptor which belongs to the G-protein-coupled receptor (GPCR) superfamily. These autoantibodies (TRAb) result in hyperthyroidism, which entails symptoms from many organs, including the heart with risk for tachyarrhythmia, atrial fibrillation and heart failure. In previous studies of GD patients with heart complications, antibodies targeting cardiovascular GPCRs including the β1-adrenergic receptor (B1R) were shown to be frequent. However, most of these studies were relatively small and used non-standardised peptide based ELISA methods or complex cell assays for antibody assessment. In this study, we used a standardised ELISA assay (CellTrend) to analyse antibodies directed against conformational B1R epitopes (B1RAb) to investigate if such antibodies are increased in GD patients compared to healthy controls, are influenced by antithyroid treatment and correlate with TRAb levels or heart related symptoms.

Methods: This is a preliminary report of results from GD patients in an ongoing longitudinal observational prospective study. Premenopausal women in profound hyperthyroidism were included and symptom scores, TRAb and B1RAb were measured at baseline and after 7.5 months of treatment. We here present results from the first enrolled 43 patients and matched controls.

Results: B1RAb levels were higher in patients at baseline compared to healthy controls (median 1.9 vs 0.9 µg/ml, $P<0.0001$). B1RAb levels decreased after 7.5 months of treatment (median 1.6 µg/ml, $P=0.001$), but remained higher than in controls ($P=0.0008$). B1RAb levels did not correlate with TRAb levels or heart related clinical symptoms.

DOI: 10.18416/RAB.2018.1809005   Advances in RAB Research • Article ID: 1809005

Conclusion: B1R autoantibodies were increased in GD patients at study inclusion and decreased with treatment. Continued studies include analysis of antibodies against other GPCRs expressed in the cardiovascular system and the relation to biomarkers of heart function.

DOI: 10.18416/RAB.2018.1809005   Advances in RAB Research • Article ID: 1809005

Infinite Science
Publishing

Patterns of 31 new autoantibodies against G-protein-coupled receptors and growth factors

H. Bittern[a], A. Carvalho-Marques[a], C. Fouodo[a], I. König[a], S. Schinke[a,*], O. Cabral-Marques[a], H. Heidecke[b], G. Riemekasten[a]

[a] University Lübeck, Germany
[b] CellTrend GmbH, Biotechnology, Luckenwalde, Germany
* Corresponding author, email: s.schinke@uksh.de

Background: Systemic sclerosis (SSc) is a rare autoimmune disease with a significant disease burden. Scl70 and centromere ab are disease specific and prognostic antibodies. Functional ab against G protein-coupled receptors (GPCR) regulate immune function and were reported in the pathogenesis of various inflammatory diseases. Objectives: We analyzed 31 ab against GPCRs in a retrospective cohort of 71 SSc sera compared to 196 sera from healthy controls (HC). Ab levels were related to disease manifestations in order to hypothesize functional ab in SSc.

Methods: SSc patients were retrospectively characterized by mRSS, organ involvement, lab tests, spirometry and imaging. 30/71 had active disease (EUSTAR activity score). Ab patterns were analyzed using new statistical approaches: factor analysis, principal component analysis (PCA), linear discriminant analysis (LDA), cluster analysis and biserial correlation.

Results: SSc subgroups (diffuse/ limited cutaneous) differ in ab levels forming separate clusters (LDA method). Moreover, latent factors group ab and clinical disease manifestations. Factor analysis reveals VEGFR2 ab and the signaling molecule YBX1 ab to be more unique with the lowest communalities. The biserial correlation shows moderate associations between ab patterns and SSc symptoms. Compared to association of ETAR ab with Raynaud's and skin sclerosis HGFR ab are inversely correlated.

Conclusions: We describe 31 new ab against GPCR and growth factors in SSc. Ab levels can be clustered by latent factors. Some ab were linked to the absence of SSc manifestations. Thus, we postulate that a dysbalance of functionally protective autoantibodies, that can be found in healthy individuals and the appearance of SSc specific ab such as Scl70 contribute to its pathogenesis. Considering the preliminary character of our data, the functional impact of ab against GPCR and growth factors has to be validated in vitro and statistical correlations to be confirmed in a prospective independent patient cohort.

DOI: 10.18416/RAB.2018.1809006   Advances in RAB Research • Article ID: 1809006

Section 3
Are anti-GPCR ab pathogenic?

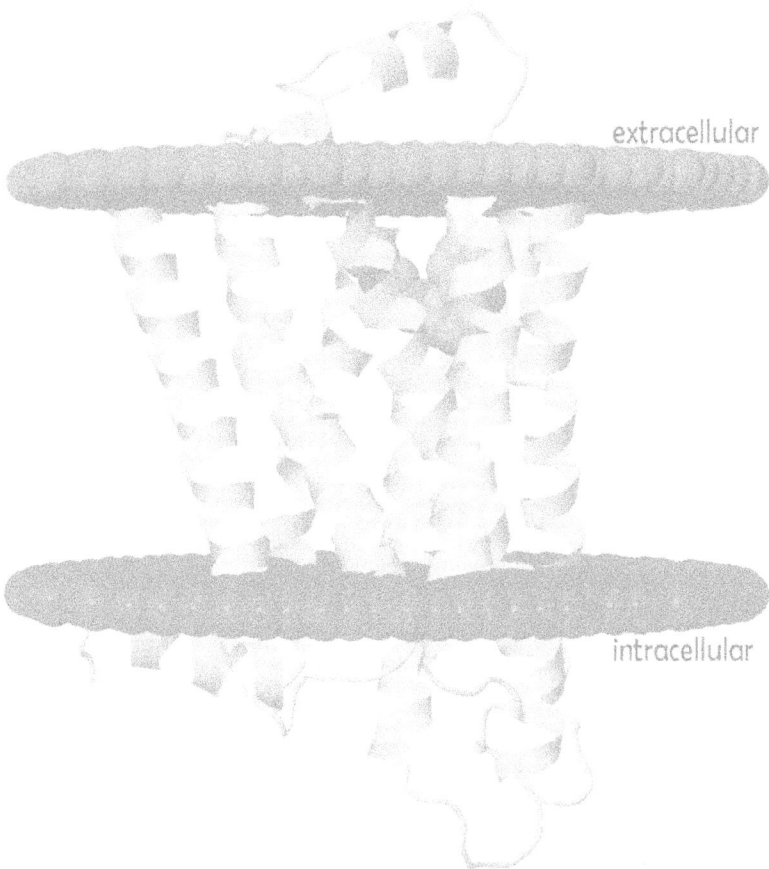

extracellular

intracellular

Diagnostics of beta-adrenergic receptor autoantibodies in chronic heart failure

Fritz Boege

Central Institute for Clinical Chemistry and Laboratory Diagnostics, Med. Faculty, Univ. Düsseldorf
Corresponding author, email: boege@uni-duesseldorf.de

Chronic heart failure (CHF) can be associated with autoantibodies targeting extracellular domains of cardiac β1-adrenergic receptors (β1AR). These auto-epitopes are related to the conformational state of the active receptor. CHF caused or promoted by such conformational β1AR autoantibodies can be ameliorated by specific therapies aimed at tolerance induction, removal or neutralisation of β1AR autoantibodies, provided the right patients are selected. Selection of such patients requires reliable detection and quantitation of circulating β1AR autoantibodies and a valid assessment of their cardio-pathogenic potential.

Reliable detection of potentially pathogenic β1AR autoantibodies can be based on IgG-binding to native β1AR presented on native cells or cell membranes, while assays using denatured cells or tissues or immobilised linear peptide mimics of the presumed auto-epitopes as antigenic targets exhibit insufficient sensitivity, most probably because epitope conformation is not or only inadequately represented. Reconstitution of the conformational epitope from composite or circular peptides is under current investigation. Assessment of the putative cardio-pathogenic potential of β1AR autoantibodies must be based on their effects on receptor function and signal transduction that are indeed causal for the development and progression of CHF. Identification of such disease-relevant functional cascades and their specific assessment in medical diagnostic will be a crucial prerequisite for the implementation of novel specific therapies not only for β1AR autoantibodies in CHF by but also for most other diseases involving autoantibodies that target G-protein-coupled receptors (GPCR).

Unfortunately, little is known about the pathways connecting IgG-binding to GPCR with the development or progression of human diseases. In the case of CHF-associated ?1AR autoantibodies it is established that the autoantibodies of the IgG type and stabilise or induce an active conformation of the β1AR. Thereby, they induce/promote CHF most notably of the iDCM type. It is clear that the pathogenic mechanism triggered by the antibodies starts with stimulation of the β1AR and ends with altered cardiomyocte contractility, electric cardiac dysfunction, cardiofibrosis, and ventricular remodelling as ultimate pathological endpoints. However, the mechanistic cascade linking these two points remains unclear. It has not even been sorted out, which cell type is the crucial primary target of the autoantibodies (i.e. β1-AR stimulation on which cell triggers the cardio-pathogenic development). Current discussions encompass down-regulation of β1AR-signaling on cardiomyocytes, β-arrestin-mediated processes in cardiomyocytes including ER-stress and apoptosis, alteration of the secretory phenotype of cardiac fibroblasts, and stimulation of IL-6 secretion in T-lymphocytes.

DOI: 10.18416/RAB.2018.1809007   Advances in RAB Research • Article ID: 1809007

Future research efforts should be directed at evaluating in longitudinal studies the various known functional effects of the autoantibodies and to develop diagnostic tests for those effects that exhibit the strongest correlation with the onset and progression of CHF, and/or provide the highest positive predictive value for the beneficial effects of antibody-directed therapies.

DOI: 10.18416/RAB.2018.1809007   Advances in RAB Research • Article ID: 1809007

Novel targets in the diagnosis of autoimmune and non-autoimmune diseases

Harald Heidecke

CellTrend GmbH, Luckenwalde, Germany
Corresponding author, email: heidecke@celltrend.de

Antibodies against GPCR are present in autoimmune and non-autoimmune diseases. Furthermore, CellTrend described for the first time antibodies against growth factors (GF, e.g. VEGF-A) and their related receptors (GFR, e.g. EGF-R). Elevated as well as decreased antibodies against GPCRs, GFs and GFRs are present in many diseases. There are a growing number of antibodies against different GPCR, GF and GFRs. The following ELISAs for the quantitative determination of AT1R-Ab, ETAR-Ab, ETBR-Ab, PAR1-Ab, PAR2-Ab, M1R-Ab, M2R-Ab, M3R-Ab, M4R-Ab, M5R-Ab, Complement-Receptor-5a-Ab, CXCR3-Ab, CXCR4-Ab, α1-adr-R-Ab, α2-adr-R-Ab, β1-adr-R-Ab, β2-adr-R-Ab, VEGF-A-Ab, VEGF-B-Ab, VEGFR1-Ab, EGF-Ab, EGFR-Ab and PlGF-Ab are available as kits. Some of these assays are registered as in vitro Diagnostica (IvD). In addition, antibodies against Serotonin-R, Dopamin-R and FGF are available as a CellTrend lab service. Current findings indicate the important role of anti-GPCR, anti-GF, anti-GFR antibody patterns as markers of diseases. Therefore, further studies determining the whole spectrum of antibodies targeting GPCRs, GFs and GFRs in healthy subjects and in different diseases are necessary. New mathematic models for the analysis of the antibody patterns are required, too.

DOI: 10.18416/RAB.2018.1809008   Advances in RAB Research • Article ID: 1809008

Anti-AT1R ab and as cause or contributor to skin fibrosis and interstitial lung disease

Xinhua Yu

Research Center Borstel, Germany
Corresponding author, email: xinhuayu@fz-borstel.de

Introduction: Systemic sclerosis (SSc) is a complex connective tissue disease which is characterized by autoimmunity, vasculopathy and fibrosis. Recent studies have suggested that autoantibodies (ab) against angiotensin II receptor I (AT1R) might play a pathogenic role in the development of SSc, which need to be further verified by animal models in vivo. However, due to the difficulties in preparation of antigens with native conformational epitopes, induction of functional aab against surface-expressed receptors is a challenging task.

Methods: We Immunized mice with membrane extracts derived from CHO cells overexpressing human AT1R (hAT1R) and evaluated the immunological and histological phenotypes in the immunized mice.

Results: The hAT1R-immunized mice developed functional autoantibodies against AT1R which are able to bind to and to activate the native receptor. Furthermore, hAT1R-immunization induced SSc-like disease symptoms including vasculopathy and interstitial inflammation in the lung as well as perivascular inflammation and fibrosis in the skin. Importantly, the SSc-like disease can be partially transferred by the serum IgG of hAT1R-immunized mice.

Conclusion: Our study provides a new animal model for SSc, which strongly supports the hypothesis of a pathogenic role of functional antibodies against AT1R in this disease.

DOI: 10.18416/RAB.2018.1809009   Advances in RAB Research • Article ID: 1809009

Monoclonal anti-AT1R ab from a SSc mouse model: evaluation of their functions

Frank Petersen

Research Center Borstel, Germany
Corresponding author, email: fpetersen@fz-borstel.de

Introduction: Monoclonal antibodies (mAbs) to GPCR which exert a functional activation of the corresponding receptors are ultimate tools to explore their physiological and pathophysiological role in autoimmune diseases. However, generation of such antibodies appears to be difficult since most of the epitopes relevant for receptor functions are present only in the native conformation of the protein, disabling immunization and detection strategies based on linear peptides.

Methods: Using an immunization strategy established for our novel SSc-mouse model with rhu AT1R derived from membrane extracts, 3 different mAb to AT1R (clone 7.1; clone 2.2b; clone 5.2a) were generated by standard hybridoma technique. Antibodies were selected by their ability to bind to the native protein and tested for their capacity to activate AT1R receptor functions in vitro and in vivo.

Results: Antibodies of all 3 clones bind to AT1R in ELISA and on epithelial cells with different affinities. In addition, clone 2.2b interacts beside AT1R also with ETAR. Moreover, mAbs derived from clone 2.2b and 5.2a induced IL-8-release in human monocytes and modulated the bead rate of myocardinal cells, both sensitive to AT1R-antagonists. Finally, mAbs of clone 7.1 and 5.2a provoked a strong infiltration of inflammatory cells and tissue swelling after local injection into the ears of mice.

Conclusions: We have generated 3 different functional mAbs to AT1R with overlapping but not identical properties. While clone 5.2a recognizes monospecifically AT1R with high affinity and induces cytokine-release as well as inflammation, binding and functions of the two other mAbs are heterogeneous. We will make use of the different properties of the mAbs to investigate the specific role of autoantibodies to AT1R and ETAR in the pathogenesis of systemic sclerosis. Moreover, the immunization strategy presented here could be useful to develop further functional antibodies directed against other GPCR.

DOI: 10.18416/RAB.2018.1809010   Advances in RAB Research • Article ID: 1809010

Transfer of PBMC from SSc patients to immunodeficient mice leads to the production of autoantibodies against AT1R and ETAR

Xiaoyang Yue[a], Yaqing Shu[a], Junie Tchudjin Magatsin[a], Xiaoqing Wang[a],
Junping Yin Marjan Ahmadi[a], Harald Heidecke[b], Brigitte Kasper[a], Xinhua Yu[a],
Frank Petersen[a,*], Gabriela Riemekasten[*]

[a] Priority Area Asthma & Allergy, Research Center Borstel, Airway Research Center North (ARCN),
Members of the German Center for Lung Research (DZL), 23845 Borstel, Germany
[b] CellTrend GmbH, Im Biotechnologiepark, 14943 Luckenwalde, Germany
[*] Corresponding authors, email: fpeters@fz-borstel.de and Gabriela.Riemekasten@uksh.de

Backgroud and objective: Systemic sclerosis (SSc) is complex autoimmune connective tissue
disease with an unclear pathogenesis. Recently, there have been accumulating evidence that
autoantibodies against some G-protein-coupled receptors (GPCR), such as angiotensin II type-
1 receptor (AT1R) and endothelin receptor type A (ETAR) contribute to the development of
SSc. In this study, we investigated autoantibodies against AT1R and ETAR as well as clinical
features in a novel humanized mouse model for SSc induced by transfer of patients PBMC.

Methods: PBMC cells from SSc patients or health donors (HD) were transferred into the Rag2-
/-Il2-/- immune deficient mice via i.p. injection. Mice were sacrificed 12 weeks after the
transfer, and blood and tissues were collected for further evaluation. Total human IgG, anti-
AT1R IgG and anti-ETAR IgG were determined in the sera of recipient mice. Skin, lung, kidney,
heart, liver and muscle were evaluated by HE staining.

Results: Compared to mice transferred with PBMC from healthy controls, mice received PBMC
from SSc patients showed significantly higher levels of both anti-AT1R and anti-ETAR IgGs.
However, levels of total human IgG in mice sera of both groups were comparable.
Furthermore, severe inflammation was observed in lung, kidney and muscle of mice received
PBMC from SSc patients, while such inflammation was not observed in control group.

Conclusions: This study demonstrates that PBMC from patients with SSc are capable to
produce autoantibodies against GPCRs and to induce inflammation in multiple organs in vivo.

Section 4

Signaling of anti-GPCR ab:
can we identify novel targets?

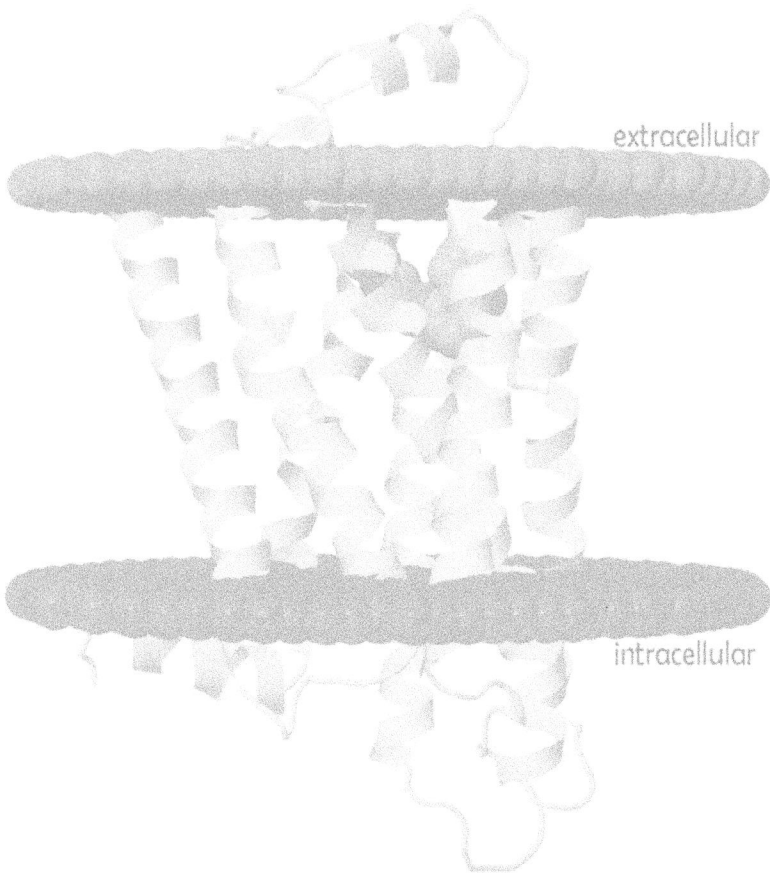

extracellular

intracellular

Infinite Science
Publishing

Signaling and GPCR biology using cell models

Philippe Aurélie

Department of Nephrology and Medical Intensive Care, CVK, Charité Universitätsmedizin Berlin
Corresponding author, email: aurelie.philippe@charite.de

A wide range of untreatable or difficult to treat disease entities are caused by activating immunoglobulins G (IgG) directed against G-protein coupled receptors (GPCR). Hence, molecular architecture of the binding of these antibodies to the receptors and the functional consequences of changes in specific structural modules are of immense clinical relevance. Our laboratory has focused over the years on the Angiotensin II type 1 receptor (AT1R) and Endothelin-1 type A receptor (ETAR), which signal upon natural ligand Angiotensin II (Ang II) or Endothelin-1 (ET-1)-mediated and AT1R- or ETAR-agonistic IgG (AT1R-/ETAR-IgG)-mediated stimulation. Development of high-resolution methods allows for structural-functional relationship studies of specific receptor modules, including the extracellular domains, in the receptor activation.

To distinguish natural peptide and IgG-mediated activation, we first developed a yeast model where human GPCR activation controls yeasts growth. These yeasts have been modified to express one single human GPCR that couples to a chimera between human and yeast G-protein. Each yeast strain is specific of a different G-protein.

Point mutations can be introduced by site-directed mutagenesis in order to determine the influence of amino acids sequences on the receptor activation. To investigate further the link between conformation and activation of the receptor in a more complicated environment, we performed luciferase reporter assays in Human Microvascular Endothelial Cells (HMEC-1) after transfecting the cells with wild type or mutated receptors and the appropriate reporter plasmids. Comparison between wild-type and mutants, non-stimulated and stimulated cells allowed us to better characterize the influence of the conformation changes on activation of the receptors.

We successfully created models allowing for structural and functional studies of molecular architecture modules appreciating GPCR receptor plasticity, which helped us to define the role of specific extracellular domains. Better understanding of the molecular mechanisms responsible for GPCR activation holds great potential for design of more specific drugs in autoantibody-mediated diseases.

Lessons from dermatology: Anti-Dsg1/3 und anti-BP180-induced signaling

Ralf Ludwig

Lübeck Inst. of Experimental Dermatology, University of Lübeck, Germany
Corresponding author, email: ralf.ludwig@uksh.de

Pemphigus and pemphigoid diseases are prototypical, organ-specific autoimmune diseases of the skin. Despite recent advances in treatment options, the morbidity and mortality of the patients remains high. Immunologically, pemphigus and pemphigoid diseases are characterized and caused by autoantibodies targeting structural proteins of the skin.

In pemphigus, autoantibodies against desmoglein (Dsg) 1 and/or 3 directly induce intraepidermal blistering – independent of the Fc fragment of the autoantibodies. While the exact mode of blistering induced by anti-Dsg1/3 is still controversially discussed, involvement of kinases in this process has been firmly established. A comprehensive overview of kinase activity is so far, however lacking. To address this knowledge gap, and to identify potential novel therapeutic targets, we evaluated the effects of a kinase-inhibitor library on Dsg-1/3-induced alterations in keratinocytes. Identified kinase inhibitors were then validated in an ex vivo full-skin thickness model of pemphigus.

In total, 5 novel kinases were identified to contribute to Dsg-1/3 autoantibody-induced blistering in pemphigus. In pemphigoid diseases, the autoimmune response is directed against hemi-desmosomal proteins. In contrast to pemphigus, sub-epidermal blistering, accompanied by inflammation occurs in pemphigoid diseases. The inflammation is triggered by Fc-depended mechanisms, including complement activation and activation of neutrophils.

However, evidence is accumulating, that in addition to Fc-mediated effects, the binding of the autoantibodies to the targets cells also contributes to blistering in pemphigoid; e.g. release of pro-inflammatory cytokines. Herein, we investigated the effects of the same kinase-inhibitor library on BP180 (the major autoantigen in the pemphigoid disease bullous pemphigoid) autoantibody-induced cytokine release. Again, several novel targets were identified and validated. Taken together, this demonstrates that binding of autoantibodies against Dsg1/3 and BP180 induces an intracellular signaling that contributes to disease pathogenies.

DOI: 10.18416/RAB.2018.1809013   Advances in RAB Research • Article ID: 1809013

Role of antibodies against PAR-1 and PAR-2 in cancer in the kidney transplant recipients

R. Catar[a,c,*], R. Carroll[b], L. Chen[a], Q. Li[a], I. Schramm[a], M. Simon[a], O. Wischnewski[a], A. Kusch[a], A. Philippe[a], D. Dragun[a,c]

[a] Department of Nephrology and Medical Intensive Care, Campus Virchow-Klinikum, Charité Berlin Germany
[b] Royal Adelaide Hospital, Centre for Experimental Transplantation - Adelaide, Australia
[c] Berlin Institute of Health, Berlin, German
* Corresponding author, email: rusan.catar@charite.de

Background: Activated angiogenesis and impaired host immune response contribute to cancer in renal transplant recipients. Induction of VEGF is crucial for neoangiogenesis in tumors. Functional autoantibodies targeting GPCRs are able to induce endothelial dysfunction. We hypothesized that autoimmune GPCR targeting process may disturb VEGF induced angiogenesis. We identified in an in vitro model PAR-1 as novel activating autoantibody target and assessed the presence of this naturally occurring blocking antibody in 20 Kidney Transplant Recipients (KTR) with and 29 KTR without metastatic cancer. In further in vitro studies, we determined the influence of IgG derived from KTR on PAR-2-dependent G-protein activation

Methods/Materials: Human endothelial cells were stimulated with IgG isolated from sera of kidney transplant recipients (KTR-IgG). Transcriptional regulation of VEGF was studied by promoter deletion assay. Transcription factor activation and binding was assessed by qRT-PCR, western blot, EMSA and cFOS knockdown. VEGF secretion was determined by ELISA. Tube formation on matrigel served to study endothelial neoangiogenic response. G-protein activation was measured by reporter assay. All 49 patients enrolled had sera for assessment of PAR antibodies (PAR-Ab) via ELISA in 2016 and at the time of transplantation.

Results: Treatment with KTR-IgG reduced ERK1/2-dependent VEGF secretion and tube formation. VEGF secretion and endothelial tube formation could be restored by pretreatment with specific PAR-1 inhibitor. KTR-IgG contributed to deregulated neoangiogenesis via reduced VEGF promoter activity and increased cFos protein expression via its binding to the VEGF promoter. Mutation of extracellular loops of PAR2 receptor increased PAR2-Ab dependent Gq11 Signalling. Levels of PAR1-Ab were statistically significantly lower pre transplant and at diagnosis in those KTR who subsequently developed cancer compared to controls without cancer.

DOI: 10.18416/RAB.2018.1809014   Advances in RAB Research • Article ID: 1809014

Conclusion: We identified the PAR-1 receptor as a new target for functional antibodies in the context of kidney transplantation and tumor angiogenesis. PAR-1 regulated angiogenesis could offer new possibilities for treatment of kidney transplants to obviate tumor angiogenesis.

DOI: 10.18416/RAB.2018.1809014   Advances in RAB Research • Article ID: 1809014

Infinite Science
Publishing

Sialylated autoantigen-reactive IgG antibodies attenuate disease development in mouse models of lupus nephritis and rheumatoid arthritis

Yannic C. Bartsch, Johann Rahmöller, Alexei Leliavski, Gina-Maria Lilienthal, Janina Petry, Marc Ehlers[*]

University of Luebeck, Luebeck, Germany
[*] Corresponding author, email: marc.ehlers@uksh.de

Pro- and anti-inflammatory effector functions of IgG antibodies (Abs) depend on their subclass and Fc glycosylation pattern. Accumulation of non-galactosylated (agalactosylated; G0) IgG Abs in the serum of rheumatoid arthritis (RA) and systemic lupus erythematosus (SLE) patients reflects severity of the diseases. In contrast, sialylated IgG Abs are responsible for anti-inflammatory effects of the intravenous immunoglobulin (IVIG; pooled human serum IgG from healthy donors), administered in high doses (2 g/kg) to treat autoimmune patients. However, whether low amounts of sialylated autoantigen-reactive IgG Abs can also inhibit autoimmune diseases has been hardly investigated. Here, we explored whether sialylated autoantigen-reactive IgG Abs can inhibit autoimmune pathology in two mouse models (Bartsch et al., Front. Immunol. 2018; 9:1183). We found that sialylated IgG autoantibodies fail to induce inflammation and lupus nephritis in a B cell receptor (BCR) transgenic lupus model, but instead are associated with lower frequencies of pathogenic Th1, Th17 and B cell responses. In accordance, the transfer of small amounts of immune complexes containing sialylated IgG Abs was sufficient to attenuate the development of nephritis. We further showed that administration of sialylated collagen type II (Col II)-specific IgG Abs attenuated the disease symptoms in a model of Col II-induced arthritis and reduced pathogenic Th17 cell and autoantigen-specific IgG Ab responses. We conclude that sialylated autoantigen-specific IgG Abs may represent a promising tool for treating pathogenic T and B cell immune responses in autoimmune diseases.

DOI: 10.18416/RAB.2018.1809015   Advances in RAB Research • Article ID: 1809015

Autoantibodies targeting complement receptors 3a and 5a are decreased in ANCA-associated vasculitis

Sebastian Klapa[a,*], Andreas Koch[b], Anja Kerstein[a], Christian Karsten[c], Harald Heidecke[d], Markus Huber-Lang[e], Peter Lamprecht[a], Gabriela Riemekasten[a], Antje Müller[a]

[a] Department of Rheumatology & Clinical Immunology, University of Lübeck & Institute for Experimental Medicine Christian-Albrechts-University Kiel c/o German Naval Medical Institute, Kronshagen, Germany
[b] Institute for Experimental Medicine Christian-Albrechts-University Kiel c/o German Naval Medical Institute, Kronshagen Germany
[c] Institute for Systemic Inflammation Research, University of Lübeck, Germany
[d] CellTrend GmbH, Luckenwalde, Germany
[e] Department of Orthopaedic, Trauma, Hand, Plastic and Reconstruction Surgery, University of Ulm
[*] Corresponding author, email: sebastian.klapa@uksh.de

Introduction: Necrotizing crescentic glomerulonephritis (NCGN) is a pathogenic hallmark of full-blown ANCA-associated vasculitis (AAV). In AAV, NCGN is characterized by scantly deposited immune complexes and involvement of the complement system. The relevance of the latter in AAV is reflected by elevated amounts of circulating C5a and, foremost, by protection from NCGN through blockade of C5aR1. In contrast, little if any is known about autoantibodies recognizing complement receptors 3a and 5a in AAV patients.

Methods: To examine the presence of autoantibodies directed against complement receptor C3a (C3aR) and C5a (C5aR1) in AAV, sera of patients with AAV [granulomatosis with polyangiitis (GPA), n=49 and microscopic polyangiitis (MPA), n=10] were measured by Elisa in comparison to healthy controls (HC, n=127). In addition, amounts of circulating C3a and C5a were determined by Elisa. Clinical parameters (BVAS, VDI, therapy) and disease marker (ESR, CRP, creatinine, anti-PR3, anti-MPO) were gathered at the time of serum sampling.

Results: Unlike MPA, in GPA lower titers of anti-C3aR were observed in comparison to HC. In addition, the concentration of anti-C5aR1 was decreased in both, GPA and MPA when compared to HC. In particular, GPA patients without a history of therapy using cyclophosphamide and/or rituximab exhibited a negative correlation between the concentration of anti-C5aR1 and the disease activity (BVAS).

Conclusion: The results may give a hint that anti-C3aR and anti-C5aR1 antibodies play distinct roles in GPA and MPA. Further, anti-C5aR1 might be of diagnostic value to monitor the clinical progress of GPA.

DOI: 10.18416/RAB.2018.1809016   Advances in RAB Research • Article ID: 1809016

Impact of regulatory (auto-)antibodies against G-protein-coupled receptors on blood pressure in women ten years after early-onset preeclampsia

Anna Birukov[a,d,e,f,g]*, Hella Muijsers[c], Harald Heidecke[b], Nadine Haase[a,d,e,f,g], Kristin Kräker[a,d,e,f,g], Dominik N. Müller[a,d,e,f,g], Florian Herse[a,d,e,f,g], Angela Maas[c], Ralf Dechend[a,d,e,f,g,h]

[a] Experimental and Clinical Research Center, a joint cooperation between Max-Delbrück-Center for Molecular Medicine and Charité - Universitätsmedizin Berlin, Corporate Member of Freie Universität Berlin, Humboldt-Universität zu Berlin, and Berlin Institute of Health, Berlin, Germany
[b] CellTrend GmbH, Luckenwalde, Germany
[c] Radboud University Medical Center, Department of Cardiology, Nijmegen, The Netherlands
[d] DZHK (German Center for Cardiovascular Research), Partner site Berlin, Berlin, Germany
[e] Charité - Universitätsmedizin Berlin, Corporate Member of Freie Universität Berlin, Humboldt-Universität zu Berlin, and Berlin Institute of Health, Berlin, Germany
[f] Max Delbrück Center for Molecular Medicine in the Helmholtz Association, Berlin, Germany
[g] Berlin Institute of Health (BIH), Berlin, Germany
[h] Department of Cardiology and Nephrology, HELIOS Klinikum Berlin, Berlin, Germany
* Corresponding author, email: anna.birukov@charite.de

Introduction: Preeclampsia (PE) is associated with an increased cardiovascular risk in later life, especially in women after early-onset PE. We and others have shown that activating antibodies against angiotensin II receptor type 1 (AT1-) are present in women with PE, even after pregnancy. Further, regulatory (auto-) antibodies against G-coupled receptors (GPCR) have been shown to contribute to cardiovascular disease.

Hypothesis: Regulatory autoantibodies' titers are elevated in women with a history of early onset PE and correlate to physiological parameters and clinical outcomes.

Methods: Autoantibodies against AT1-, β1- adrenergic receptors, endothelin I receptor A (ETAR), protease-activated receptor 1 (PAR1) and C-X-C3 chemokine binding receptors (CXCR3) were determined by using commercially available ELISA (Celltrend, Luckenwalde, Germany) in women 10 years after after PE pregnancy or control pregnancy. We investigated samples from the PREVFEM cohort (PReeclampsia Risk EValuation in FEMales), a retrospective matched case-control study, which was performed in Zwolle, The Netherlands, from 2008 until 2010. All women registered in the early preeclampsia database as well as an equal number of age-matched females without preeclampsia from the regular obstetric database in the same time period (1991-2007) were invited to participate in the PREVFEM study.

DOI: 10.18416/RAB.2018.1809017   Advances in RAB Research • Article ID: 1809017

Results: Women with history of early PE had higher prevalence of hypertension than controls (42.7% vs 8.3%, p < 0.001). Women with the lowest combined levels of autoantibodies and a history of early PE had significantly higher SBP (mean difference = 11.54 mmHg, 95% CI [4.39; 18.70], p < 0.001), DBP (mean difference = 7.75 mmHg, 95% CI [2.42; 13.08], p < 0.001), and MAP (mean difference = 9.02 mmHg, 95% CI [3.24; 14.79], p < 0.001) compared to the controls. The titer levels of single regulatory AT1-, β1-, ETAR-, PAR1- and CXCR3-autoantibodies were not different between control and former PE women 10 years after index pregnancy.

Conclusions: Hypertension is a common problem after preeclamptic pregnancy in middle-aged women. Regulatory autoantibodies are not sufficient alone to cause hypertension or other pathologic conditions, but together with other risk factors such as pathological pregnancy might drive the whole balance towards pathophysiologic conditions. Further studies are needed to investigate the potential of regulatory autoantibodies against GPCR as pre-symptomatic biomarkers identifying women at particular cardiovascular risk.

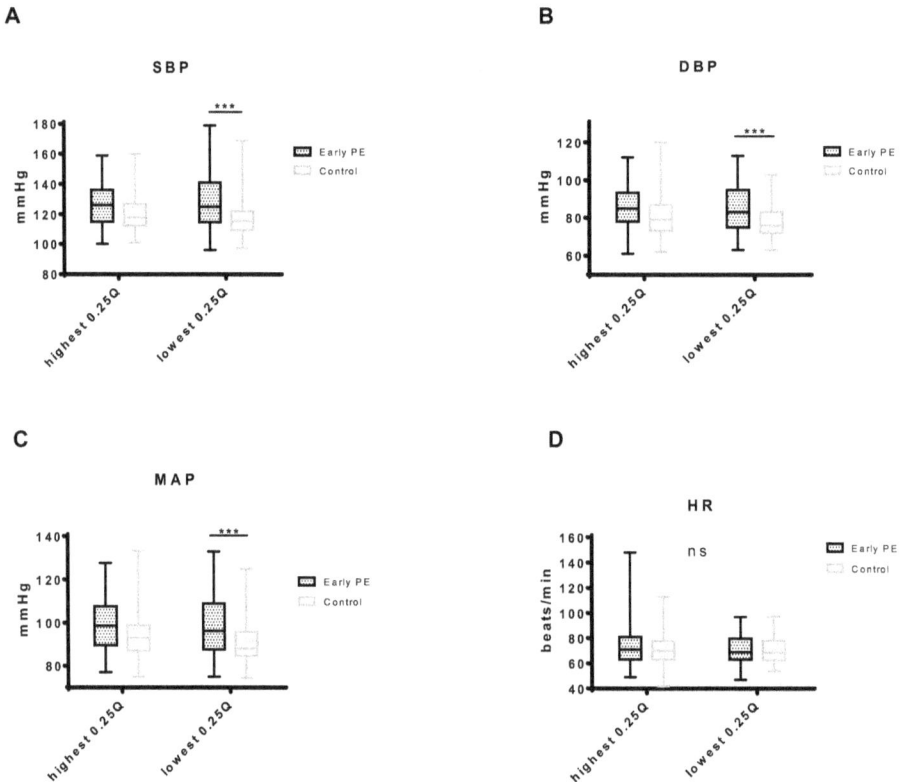

Figure 1. Systolic (A), diastolic (B) blood pressure, mean arterial pressure (C) and heart rate (D) in women with the highest vs. lowest total levels of autoantibodies, stratified by the pregnancy outcome. Highest 0.25Q = upper 0.25 quantile, lowest 0.25 quantile of autoantibodies levels. Comparisons were performed by the Mann-Whitney U-test.

Section 5

Anti-GPCR ab as marker for diseases and therapeutic responses

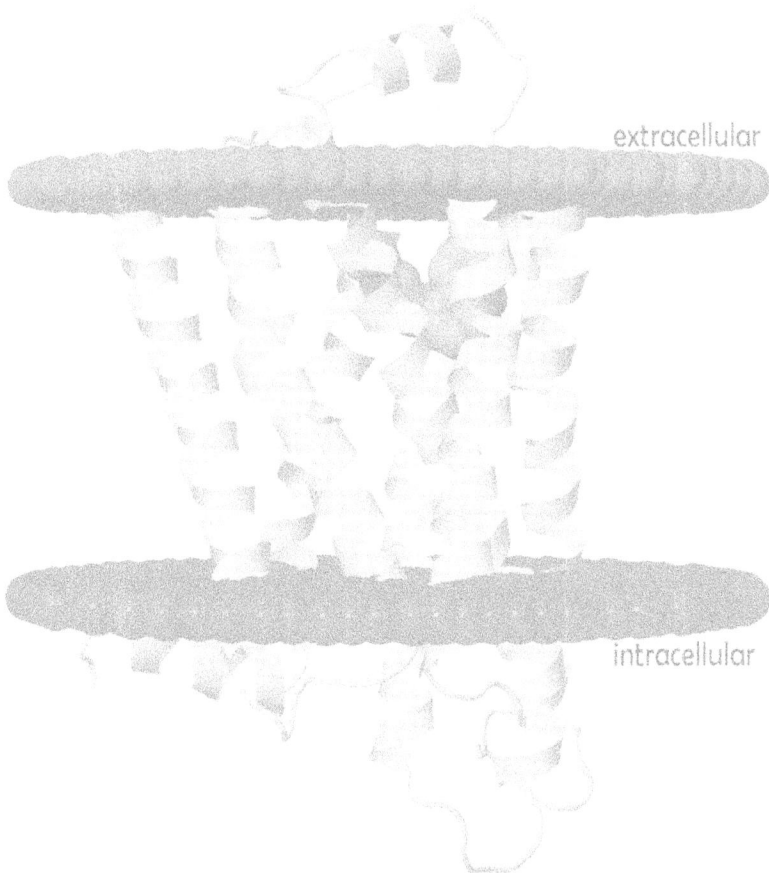

extracellular

intracellular

Antibodies against complement receptors: impact on pathophysiology

Christian Karsten

Institut für Systemische Entzündungsforschung (ISEF), Universität zu Lübeck, Germany,
Corresponding author, email: Christian.Karsten@uksh.de

Complement activation and in particular the generation of the anaphylatoxin C5a is an important mechanism of the innate immune system in response to danger signals, which compromise the integrity of the host. C5a/C5a receptor 1 (C5aR1) interactions are causing infiltration and activation of several immunologic cell types and the secretion of pro-inflammatory mediators. However, self-reactive IgGs can induce detrimental inflammation in autoimmune diseases such as systemic lupus erythematosus, rheumatoid arthritis or epidermolysis bullosa acquisita (EBA) involving unwanted activation of the complement system. Regulation of complement activation through soluble and receptor-bound complement regulatory proteins such as factor H, CD46, CD55, CD59 is well appreciated.

However, less is known about the regulation of anaphylatoxins and their induced effects. Previously, we could show that highly galactosylated IgG1 IC (Hi-Gal IC) cross-link the inhibitory IgG receptor FcγRIIB and the C-type lectin-like receptor Dectin-1 to suppress C5a-mediated effector functions in vitro and in vivo. More specifically, we found that the FcγRIIB/Dectin-1 cross-linking induces a signaling cascade driving the phosphorylation of Src homology 2 domain containing inositol phosphatase (SHIP) downstream of FcγRIIB, which in turn blocked C5aR1-mediated ERK1/2 phosphorylation. Importantly, using such Hi-Gal IC in an experimental mouse model of EBA, a subepidermal autoimmune blistering disease, resulted in a significant reduction of the disease phenotype. Interestingly, in the serum of patients with scleroderma we found auto-antibodies against C5aR1, which have the same therapeutic potential as Hi-Gal IC. These anti-C5aR1 antibodies are able to directly inhibit C5a/C5aR1-mediated effector functions, suggesting, that these intrinsic auto-antibodies produced alongside with other auto-antibodies might play important roles in the regulation of innate and adaptive immune responses in scleroderma.

DOI: 10.18416/RAB.2018.1809018   Advances in RAB Research • Article ID: 1809018

Anti-GPCR antibodies in atherosclerosis

Zouhair Aherrahrou[a,*], Laurence Johanson[b], Jeanette Erdmann[a], Gabriela Riemekasten[b]

[a] Institute for Cardiogenetics, Universität zu Lübeck; DZHK (German Centre for Cardiovascular Research), Partner Site Hamburg/Kiel/Lübeck, Germany; University Heart Centre Lübeck, 23562 Lübeck, Germany
[b] Department of Rheumatology, Universität zu Lübeck, Lübeck, Germany
[*] Corresponding author, email: zouhair.aherrahrou@uni-luebeck.de

Cardiovascular diseases, including coronary artery disease (CAD), are considered as killer number one worldwide. The pathology of CAD is caused by atherosclerosis, an inflammatory and immunological disorder. CXCL12 has been reported to be associated with CAD by genome-wide association studies (GWAS) and thus the CXCL12 / CXCR4 axis is determinant in atherosclerosis. CXCR4 belongs to the G proteins-coupled receptors (GPCR), which modulate different cellular functions. Although GPCRs are well established to function in immunity and inflammation, a little is known about their exact role in atherosclerosis. Recent studies pinpointed their therapeutic potential for atherosclerosis and CAD, however strong pre-clinical experimental evidence is still missing to understand whether targeting each of those molecules is protective or detrimental for atherosclerosis.

Here we will provide a short update on the so far published data with regard to the potential implication of both receptors CXCR3 and 4 as well their ligands CXCL9-12 in the context of atherosclerosis. Recently a high anti-CXCR3/4 antibodies in patients with systemic sclerosis (SSc) along with other GPCRs was reported. An attempt to treat atherogenic mice with IgGs from systemic sclerosis (SSc) patients and healthy controls (HC) is in progress. Some of the so far generated preliminary results will be presented and discussed. This update will help us to further extend our better understanding on targeting GPCRs in the context of atherosclerosis.

Immunoadsorption in Vascular Dementia - a novel approach to Alzheimer´s Disease?

Hans Jörgen Grabe

Department of Psychiatry and Psychotherapy, University of Greifswald, Greifswald, Germany
Corresponding author, email: grabeh@uni-greifswald.de

The pathomechanisms leading to Alzheimer´s Disease (AD) are not well understood. Despite several robust hypotheses the nature of the disease seems to be more complex than initially thought. The role of vascular components of AD have been underestimated so far. In this novel treatment approach we perform immunoadsorption over 5 days to remove agonistic autoantibodies (AAB) against α1A-adrenoceptor from the plasma of AD patients. These AAB are thought to alter the functional properties of small blood vessels leading to malfunctions in the supply and clearance processes of the brain.

We will present the first 5 patients with AD who underwent immunoabsorption and who completed a 12-months follow up. Clinical, cognitive and MRI data as well as peripheral endothelial function data and data on AAB clearance will be presented.

The study is funded by Fresenius Medical Care.

First results of the prospective ETiCS-study: acute (microbial-associated) inflammation rather than (infarction-associated) myocardial ischemia triggers the development of cardiac GPCR autoantibodies

Valérie Boivin-Jahns[a], Chistina Zechmeister[a], Claudia Schuetz[a], Niklas Beyersdorf[b], Stefan Stoerk[c], Roland Jahns[d,*]

[a] Institute of Pharmacology and Toxicology, University Wuerzburg, Germany
[b] Institute of Immunobiology, University Wuerzburg, Germany
[c] Comprehensive Heart Failure Center, University Hospital Wuerzburg, Germany
[d] Interdisciplinary Bank of Bio-materials and Data Wuerzburg , University and University Hospital Wuerzburg, Germany
[*] Corresponding author, email: Jahns_r@ukw.de

Introduction: Heart failure (HF) is the leading cause of mortality and morbidity in developed countries. In the past decade evidence for a clinical relevance of GPCR-autoimmunity in human HF has substantially increased. Stimulating autoantibodies targeting the second extracellular loop (ECII) of the cardiac beta1-adrenoceptor (beta1-aabs) have been claimed to be involved in the pathogenesis of HF and to increase the risk of cardio-vascular death by three-fold. Still, the events triggering the formation of beta1-aabs and their impact on HF-progression are unknown.

Methods: Based on the rationale that presentation of beta1-adrenoceptors and other cardiac membrane antigens following inflammation or necrosis may induce the formation of beta1-aabs, in total 13 University Hospitals (12 in Germany, 1 in Serbia) prospectively recruited 226 patients with a first acute myocardial infarction (FAMI), and 140 pts with acute (biopsy- or cMRI-proven) myocarditis (AMitis) into the Etiology, Titer-Course and effect on Survival of cardiac autoantibodies-study (ETiCS-study). At baseline (BL) and three follow-up visits (Fup1-3) blood was sampled to follow the time-course of various GPCR-aabs. Beta1-aabs were assessed by using Dynabeads® M-270-Epoxy coated with increasing amounts of beta1-ECII-peptides (2.5-100 µg/ml). As control, beads were coated with a peptide comprising same amino-acids, but in a scrambled order. After reacting with the beads (15min on ice) the samples were measured on a FACScan flow-cytometer. Data were analyzed using FlowJo (Treestar); when half-maximal binding was calculable the serum was classified beta1-aab-positive.

Results: From n=366 pts (226 FAMI/140 AMitis) recruited into the ETiCS-study 45 pts had to be excluded because of unperformed cMRI's; 46 pts stopped the study before Fup-1 (month 3). Only 180/226 FAMI- and 98/140 AMitis-pts had complete Fup1-3 (after 3, 6, and 12 months, including clinical evaluation, echocardiograms, and cMRI's at BL & Fup-3). All valid ETiCS-pts (197 FAMI-/123 AMitis-pts) were assessed for the formation of beta1-aabs, and then compared focussed on the development of echo-LVEF. In the course of the study relevant (high-affinity) beta1-aab-titres were detected in ~31% (37/123) of the AMitis-pts compared to only ~21% (42/197) of the FAMI-pts. In aab-positive AMitis-pts echo-LVEF did not recover and was always significantly inferior to aab-negative AMitis-pts (BL: 38 vs. 49% LVEF; Fup-3: 49 vs. 64% LVEF) whereas such a difference was not noted in FAMI-pts. In addition, aab-positive AMitis-pts had higher NT pro-BNP-, renin-, and aldosterone-levels than aab-negative AMitis-pts.

Conclusion: These first results from the ETiCS-study suggest that acute microbial-induced rather than post-infarction myocardial inflammation triggers the formation of clinically relevant beta1-aabs. AAb-positive AMitis-patients might profit from early intensification of standard HF-therapy (including early beta-blockade) and/or novel antibody-directed experimental therapies which are currently under development.

Section 6

How to target effects of functional antibodies

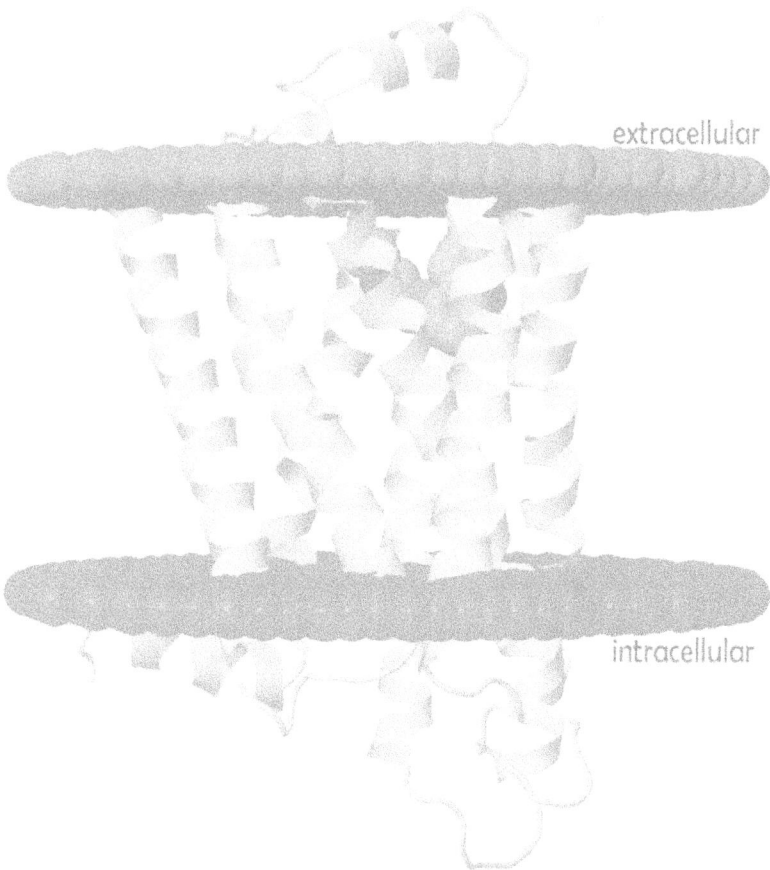

extracellular

intracellular

Immunoadsorption to remove ß adrenergic and M acetylcholine receptor antibodies in Chronic Fatigue Syndrome (CFS/ME)

Carmen Scheibenbogen[a,e,*], Markus Tölle[b] Antonia Berz[a], Helma Freitag[a], Franziska Sotzny[a], Wolfram Doehner[c], Nadja Scherbakov[c], Sandra Bauer[a], Michaela Antelmann[a], Harald Heidecke[d], Patricia Grabowski[a]

[a] Institute for Medical Immunology, Charité Berlin
[b] Department of Nephrology, Charité
[c] Center for Stroke Research Berlin, Charité
[d] CellTrend GmbH, Luckenwalde, Germany
[e] Berlin-Brandenburg Center for Regenerative Therapies (BCRT), Charité.
[*] Corresponding author, email: carmen.scheibenbogen@charite.de

Background: Infection-triggered disease onset, chronic immune activation and autonomic dysregulation in CFS/ME point to an autoimmune disease directed against neurotransmitter receptors. We observed elevated autoantibodies against ß2 adrenergic, and muscarinic (M) 3 and 4 acetylcholine receptors in a subset of patients (Löbel 2016). Immunoadsorption (IA) was shown to be effective in removing autoantibodies and to improve outcome in various autoimmune diseases.

Methods: 10 patients with post-infectious CFS/ME with elevated ß2 adrenergic, some also with M 3/4 acetylcholine receptor antibodies were treated with IA with an IgG-binding column (Globaffin, Fresenius) for 5 days followed by 25g IVIG. As outcome parameter severity of symptoms were assessed by questionnaires, autoantibodies were determined by ELISA and the B cell phenotype characterized by flow cytometry. 5 patients who improved after IA received a 2nd modified IA course to improve tolerability.

Results: Serum IgG levels dropped below median 1g/l (normal 7-16g/l) after the 5th IA, while IgA and IgM levels remained unchanged. Similarly, elevated IgG autoantibodies rapidly decreased during IA in 9 of 10 patients. Also 6 months later ß2 autoantibodies were significantly lower compared to pretreatment. Frequency of memory B cells significantly decreased and frequency of plasma cells increased after the 4th IA cycle. A rapid improvement of symptoms was reported by 7 patients during the IA. 3 of these patients had long lasting moderate to marked improvement for more than 24 months, 2 patients had short improvement only and 2 patients improved for several months following initial worsening. During treatment several patients had transient worsening of fatigue towards the end of treatment. 5 patients (2 with ongoing improvement, 3 who had relapsed) received a 2nd IA treatment with a modified schedule with improved tolerability.

Conclusions: Autoantibodies against ß adrenergic and M acetylcholine receptor can be effectively removed by IA and several patients had rapid improvement of symptoms. B cell phenotyping provides evidence for alteration of memory B cells by IA.

The aptamer BC 007 completely neutralizes agonistic autoantibodies directed against β1-adrenoceptors: Results of a phase 1 trial

Niels-Peter Becker*, Johannes Mueller, Annekathrin Haberland, Katrin Wenzel,
Gerd Wallukat, Peter Goettel, Sarah Schulze- Rothe, Ingolf Schimke, Georg Golor,
Matthias Grossmann, Angela Sinn, Martina Steiper, Tuba Yilmaz, Anne Wallukat,
Hanna Davideit, Susanne Becker

Berlin Cures, Berlin, Germany, Parexel, Berlin, Germany
* Corresponding author, email: becker@berlincures.de

Background: 80 percent of patients with non-ischemic heart failure (HF) and reduced ejection fraction have autoantibodies against β1- adrenoceptors (β1-AAB), which cause and/or sustain HF. The removal of β1-AAB by immunoadsorption (IA) leads to an improvement of cardiac function and significantly reduced mortality. With the aptamer BC 007, a new drug is under study that neutralizes autoantibodies against G-Protein-coupled receptors (GP-AAB) including β1-AAB. Aptamers are often referred to as "chemical antibodies" and offer a number of advantages over e.g. peptides and biologics when used for treatment. Based on in vitro studies followed by animal testing, BC 007 was recently step-by-step transferred to humans. We present here a Phase I study investigated the safety, tolerability, and pharmacological effect of BC 007.

Methods: In a randomized, double blind, placebo controlled single ascending dose study, 3 cohorts of 8 male healthy subjects each (age 18 - 45 yrs) were dosed with 15, 50 and 150 mg of BC 007 by i. v. infusion over 20 min. Additional 8 elderly healthy subjects of both sexes (55 - 70 yrs) received 150 mg BC007 or placebo. Subsequently, in an open labelled study part with 5 cohorts of 6 elderly volunteers each (55 - 75 yrs), who showed evidence for GP-AAB dosages of 50, 150, 300, 450, and 750 mg were tested. Infusion duration was 20 min in the 50 and 150 mg and 40 min in the 300, 450 and 750 mg cohort. Subjects safety was carefully monitored during the study (ECG, blood pressure, lab, injection site reactions, VS, physical examination, adverse events). 12 blood samples were taken from before the infusion began until 24 h thereafter for clinical chemistry, hematological and pharmacokinetic analysis. Urine was collected.

DOI: 10.18416/RAB.2018.1809023   Advances in RAB Research • Article ID: 1809023

Results: BC 007 was extremely well tolerated and without clinically relevant adverse events. GP-AAB neutralization has been seen 24 h after BC 007 infusion in 1 of 6 individuals in the 150 mg cohort, in 2/6 in the 300 and 400 mg and 5/6 in the 750 mg cohort. A slightly elevated aPTT (max 49 s) was observed in 5 subjects of the 300, 450, and 750 mg cohort which quickly normalized after end of infusion. AUC increased by rising dosage from 21 to 556 µg*min/mL, Cmax increased from 1610 to 15832 ng/mL. The half-life was short at appr 4 min.

Conclusion: BC 007 is a powerful new drug for the neutralization of β1-AAB with a favorable side-effect profile which will be tested as the first causative acting drug for patients with β1-AAB induced heart failure. Derived from IA data, a huge number of patients with HF will profit from this new drug.

Agonistic antibody diseases = Autoimmune diseases? From bench to bedside

R. Kunze

Science Office Immunology, 13125 Berlin, Germany
Corresponding author, email: Rudolf.Kunze@gmx.de

In recent years, the number of diseases in which autoantibodies (AAB) against G Protein-coupled receptors (GPCR) have been detected has continued to increase. Because they act in a bioassay similar to the physiological ligands of GPCR, the term "agonistic autoantibodies" (agAAB) was established early on. The proportion of patients with a clinically diagnosed disease in whom agAAB has been detected in the blood can be very different. Currently agAAB can be determined against 8 different GPCRs. The probably most important ones are directed against the adrenoceptors (AR) α, ß1, ß2 and the angiotensin2 receptor type 1 (AT1-R). The AAB binding epitopes are located on the extracellular 1st or 2nd loop and are consistently constant.

For a few diseases such as dilated cardiomyopathy (DCM, ß1-AR, α-AR), pre-eclampsia (AT1-R) and vascular necrotic kidney transplant rejection (AT1-R), antibodies could be induced in animal experiments by immunisation with the extracellular loop peptides and subsequently produce a disease pattern similar to that of humans. In the development of vascular M. Alzheimer's disease (VAD), animal experimental findings according to agAAK against α-AR could also play a role in cerebral vascular obliteration. For most of the diseases associated with agAAB, the pathological significance of the proven agAAB has not yet been clarified. They may be an epiphenomenon, but can also be pathologically amplifying bystander or even cause the disease.

The above agAABs often occur in typical combinations, and we do not yet know anything about their possible interference or parallel involvement in the respective disease. The distribution patterns of agAAK in diseases such as DCM, VAD, diabetes type 2 (DM2), primary open-angle glaucoma (POAG), thromboangiitis obliterans (TAO) or chronic fatigue syndrome (CFS) observed so far suggest that there are pathophysiological similarities between the very different diseases in the clinical symptoms. This is particularly noticeable in diseases with vascular contribution.

Up to now, agAAB's participation in a disease beyond the classics such as DCM has not been taken into account therapeutically. The abundance of data on the prevalence of agAAB in a wide variety of diseases makes it almost necessary to search for new terms to take these conditions into account. One possible approach would be to label patients with different diagnoses and positive antibody status with the additional diagnosis"agonistic antibody disease". In specific individual cases, new therapeutic options may then become apparent.

DOI: 10.18416/RAB.2018.1809024   Advances in RAB Research • Article ID: 1809024

Autoantibodies in serum of systemic scleroderma patients: peptide-based epitope mapping indicates increased binding to cytoplasmic domains of CXCR3

Andreas Recke[a], Ann-Katrin Regensburger[b],*, Florian Weigold[c], Antje Müller[d], Harald Heidecke[e], Gabriele Marschner[d], Christoph M. Hammers[a], Ralf J. Ludwig[b], Gabriela Riemekasten[b]

[a] Department of Dermatology, University of Lübeck, Lübeck, Germany
[b] Lübeck Institute of Dermatological Research, University of Lübeck, Lübeck, Germany
[c] Dept. of Rheumatology and Clinical Immunology, Charité University Hospital, Berlin, Germany
[d] Dept. of Rheumatology, University of Lübeck, Lübeck, Germany
[e] CellTrend GmbH, Luckenwalde, Berlin, Germany
* Corresponding author, email: Ann-Katrin.Regensburger@gmx.de

Introduction: Systemic sclerosis (SSc) is a severe chronic autoimmune disease with high morbidity and mortality. Sera of patients with SSc contain a large variety of autoantibody (aab) reactivities. Among these are functionally active aab that bind to G protein-coupled receptors (GPCR) such as C-X-C motif chemokine receptor 3 (CXCR3) and 4 (CXCR4). Aab binding to the N-terminal portion of these two GPCRs have been shown to be associated with slower disease progression in SSc, especially deterioration of lung function.

Methods: We used peptide ELISA with serum samples in combination with a hierarchical Bayesian model for mapping of epitopes on CXCR3. For in silico prediction of epitopes on CXCR3, we used the ABCpred online tool.

Results: To identify linear epitopes of anti-CXCR3 aabs, we used a peptide array of 36 overlapping 18-20mer peptides covering the entire CXCR3 sequence for ELISA to compare the binding pattern of SSc patient sera (N=32) and healthy controls (N=30). We found increased binding of SSc patient sera to intracellular epitopes within CXCR3, while the binding signal to extracellular portions of CXCR3 was found to be reduced in Ssc patients. Experimentally determined epitopes showed a good correspondence to those predicted by the ABCpred tool. To verify these results and to translate them into a novel diagnostic ELISA, we combined the peptides that represent SSc-associated epitopes into a single ELISA and evaluated its potential to discriminate SSc patients (N=31) from normal healthy controls (N=47). This ELISA had a sensitivity of 0.61 and a specificity of 0.85.

Conclusions: The clinical relevance of anti-CXCR3 aabs may crucially depend on epitope specificity, with SSc sera preferentially binding to intracellular epitopes, while healthy control sera appear to recognize an extracellular epitope in the N-terminal domain. Moreover, we propose an ELISA that could detect intracellularly binding anti-CXCR3 aabs for the monitoring of Ssc patients.

DOI: 10.18416/RAB.2018.1809025   Advances in RAB Research • Article ID: 1809025

Detection and functional characterization of angiotensin receptor Type 1 autoantibodies: establishment and clinical translation

Valérie Boivin-Jahns[a,*], Chistina Zechmeister[a], Claudia Schuetz[a], Martin J. Lohse[b],
Roland Jahns[c], Xinhua Yu[d], Frank Petersen[d], Stefanie Hahner[e], Martin Fassnacht[e]

[a] Institute of Pharmacology and Toxicology, University Wuerzburg, Germany
[b] Max-Delbrück-Centrum für Molekulare Medizin, MDC Berlin, Germany
[c] Interdisciplinary Bank of Biomaterials and Data Wuerzburg , University and University Hospital
Wuerzburg, Germany
[d] Priority Area Asthma and Allergy, Research Center Borstel, Borstel, Germany
[e] Department of Internal Medicine I, Endocrinology, University Hospital Wuerzburg, Germany
* Corresponding author, email: valerie.jahns@toxi.uni-wuerzburg.de

Introduction: Circulating AT1R autoantibodies (AT1R-aabs) directed against the ECL2 of the
AT1R with agonist-like activity are supposed to play a pathophysiological role in diseases
associated with vascular and renal damage, such as preeclampsia and malignant
hypertension (HT), but they are also thought to be involved in heart failure and primary
hyperaldosteronism (PHA).

Methods: High-throughput screening assays aiming at a reliable detection of AT1R-aabs in
sera from patients with HT and PHA were established. The agonist-like activity of AT1R-aabs
was assessed by changes in intracellular calcium levels using Fura2-QBT dye and AlphaLISA
SureFire Ultra Assay was used to assess induction of ERK1/2 phosphorylation in stably
transfected AT1R-HEK-cells.

Results: IgG purified from sera of n=60 patients with PHA and n=97 with hypertensive heart
disease (HT) were screened for their capacity to increase [Ca2+]i or to activate ERK1/2. Ten
out of 60 PHA patients increased [Ca2+]i compared to none of the HT-patients, whereas in
both disease-entities we detected AT1R-aabs inducing ERK1/2 activation with similar
prevalence (PHA: 38%, HT: 31%), indicating the existence of differentially acting AT1R-aabs.
PHA-patients positive for ERK1/2 activating AT1R-aabs have lower serum potassium- and
renin-levels together with an increased aldosterone concentration concordant with the
disease phenotype. Similarly, higher BP values (syst/diast) are observed in AT1R-aab positive
HT patients. In addition, ERK1/2-activation induced by either angiotensin II, a mouse AT1R-
Mab, or by IgG isolated from patients with PHA or HT could be differentially blocked by the
use of various signaling inhibitors. Whereas clinically used AT1R-blockers as e.g. Losartan,
Olmesartan, or Candesartan fully block Ang II-mediated ERK activation, they are less efficient
in blocking the effects of human AT1R-aabs, with Losartan having almost no effect.

DOI: 10.18416/RAB.2018.1809026   Advances in RAB Research • Article ID: 1809026

Conclusion: As hypothesized, the detection of AT1R-aabs directed against the native AT1R based on antigen binding only results in a high number of misleading results. By contrast, functional assays based on AT1R-activation ([Ca2+]i & ERK1/2-phosphorylation) are able to detect AT1R-aabs in 31% or 38% of patients with HT or PHA, respectively.

DOI: 10.18416/RAB.2018.1809026   Advances in RAB Research • Article ID: 1809026

Section 7
Posters

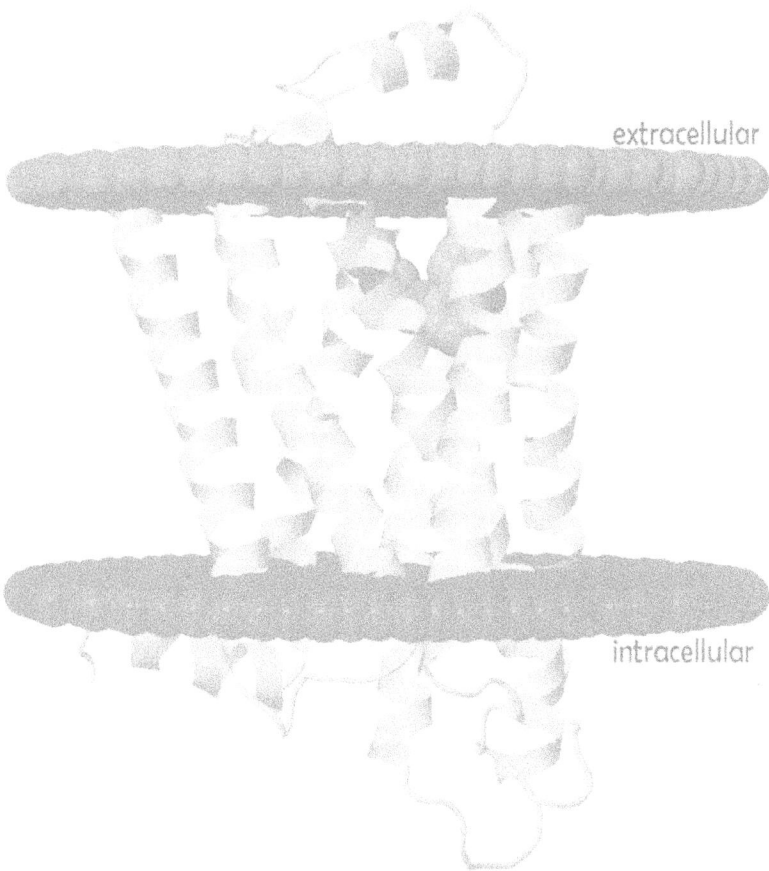

extracellular

intracellular

Autoantibodies targeting G-protein-coupled receptors in RA and SLE

Xiaoyang Xiaoyang[a,*], Qiaoniang Huang[b], Fengyuan Deng[c], Fengyuan Deng[d], Juan Chen[e], Harald Heidecke[f], Gabriela Riemekasten[g], Frank Petersen[a], Xinhua Yu[a]

[a] *Priority Area Asthma & Allergy, Research Center Borstel, Airway Research Center North (ARCN), Members of the German Center for Lung Research (DZL), 23845 Borstel, Germany*
[b] *Xiamen-Borstel Joint Laboratory of Autoimmunity, Medical College of Xiamen University, Xiamen, 361102, China*
[c] *Institute of Psychiatry and Neuroscience, Xinxiang Medical University, XinXiang, China*
[d] *Department of Rheumatology of the First Afflict Hospital of Xiamen University, Xiamen, 361003, China*
[e] *Eye Institute and Affiliated Xiamen Eye Center of Xiamen University, Xiamen, 361102, China*
[f] *CellTrend GmbH, Im Biotechnologiepark, 14943 Luckenwalde, Germany*
[g] *Department of Rheumatology, University of Lübeck, 23538, Lübeck, Germany*
* Corresponding author, email: xinhuayu@fz-borstel.de

Introduction: Previous studies have suggested a role of autoantibodies against G-protein-coupled receptors (GPCR) in autoimmune diseases. In this study, we aimed to determine the association of anti-GPCR autoantibodies with RA and SLE.

Methods: The discovery cohort consisted of 10 patients with rheumatoid arthritis (RA), 10 patients with systemic lupus erythematosus (SLE), and 10 sex- and age-matched healthy donors (HD). Serum levels of autoantibodies against 14 GPCRs were measured for the discovery cohort by ELISA (Celltrend, Germany). Autoantibodies with significant difference between patients and controls were further investigated in a validation cohort containing 40 patients with RA, 14 patients with SLE, and 40 HD. For autoantibodies confirmed in the validation cohort, bioinformatic analysis was performed to explore possible functional interactions among them, and their diagnosis values were evaluated by ROC analysis.

Results: For RA, levels of autoantibodies against 8 GPCRs were significantly different between patients and controls, 7 of which were confirmed in the validation cohort, including C5aR, C3aR, CXCR3, CXCR4, M3R, β1-adrenergic receptor and AT1R. For SLE, levels of autoantibodies against 2 GPCRs, β2-adrenergic receptor and ETAR, were significantly different between patients and controls, both were confirmed in the validation cohort. For the autoantibodies that were significantly changed in RA patients, bioinformatic analysis revealed that they were functionally related to chemotaxis. The ROC analysis showed good diagnostic values for all of those autoantibodies which were significantly changed in RA or SLE compared with controls.

Conclusion: Levels of autoantibodies against GPCRs are significantly changes in RA and SLE compared to healthy controls, suggesting that they might be associated with the development of diseases.

Identification and characterization of cytomegalovirus-specific CD8+ T cells in systemic sclerosis

Gesa Balsen[a,*], Antje Müller[a], Silke Pitann[a], Kerstin Mosenthin[a], Stoyan Dimitrov[b], Gabriela Riemekasten[a], Tanja Lange[a]

[a] Department of Rheumatology & Clinical Immunology, University of Lübeck, Germany
[b] Institut für Medizinische Psychologie und Verhaltensneurobiologie, Eberhard Karls Universität Tübingen, Tübingen, Germany
* Corresponding author, email: gesba@gmx.de

Introduction: The pathogenesis of systemic sclerosis (SSc) is linked to cytomegalovirus (CMV) infection, for instance through infected endothelial cells or via molecular mimicry inducing an autoimmune response. Further, in SSc endothelial damage might be mediated by adhesion of CMV-specific T cells. We hypothesize that CMVA2-specific CD8+ T cells display increased adhesive properties in limited and diffuse SSc, characterized by enhanced expression of CX3CR1 and activation of ?2-integrins.

Methods: Peripheral blood and serum was obtained from patients with SSc (diffuse, n=10, limited, n=10) and age-and gender-matched healthy controls (HC, n=10) and checked for HLA-A*02.01 expression due to the CMVA2 nonapeptide used. Peripheral blood mononuclear cells (PBMC) from HLA-A*02.01+ SSc patients and HC were isolated using Ficoll gradient and T lymphocytes were phenotyped (CD4, CD8, CD45RA, CCR7, CX3CR1, binding of ICAM-1 multimers) by flow cytometry. Soluble fractalkine was measured by ELISA.

Results: The frequency of CMVA2-specific CD8+ T cells was increased in diffuse SSc in comparison to both limited SSc and HC. There was no difference between SSc and HC regarding the activation of LFA-1 by CMVA2-specific CD8+ T cells. However, the expression of CX3CR1 by CMVA2-specific CD8+ T cells was elevated in SSc when compared to HC. Further, in both HC and SSc CMVA2-specific CD8+ T cells differed from non-CMV-specific CD8+ T cells with respect to the activation of LFA-1 and the expression of CX3CR1. In addition, the concentration of soluble fractalkine was higher in SSc when compared to HC.

Conclusion: An expansion of adhesive CMVA2-specific CD8+ T cells might contribute to the pathogenesis especially in diffuse SSc and should therefore be addressed therapeutically.

DOI: 10.18416/RAB.2018.1809028   Advances in RAB Research • Article ID: 1809028

Organotropism of anti-CXCR3/4- and anti-ETAR/-AT1R-mediated leukocyte migration in inflammatory and autoimmune disease

Laurence Johanson[a,*], Antje Müller[a], Zouhair Aherrahrou[b], Jennifer Hundt[c], Anja Kerstein[a], Gabriele Marschner[a], Silke Pitann[a], Sara Comdühr[a], Gesche Weppner[a], Harald Heidecke[d], Peter Lamprecht[a] , Christiane Herden[e], Gabriela Riekemasten[a]

[a] Department of Rheumatology and clinical Immunology, University Medical Center Schleswig-Holstein, Lübeck, Germany)
[b] Institute for cardiogenetics, University of Lübeck, Lübeck, Germany
[c] Dermatology, University of Lübeck, Lübeck, Germany
[d] CellTrend GmbH, Luckenwalde, Germany
[e] Institute of Veterinary Pathology, Justus-Liebig-University, Gießen, Germany
* Corresponding author, email: Laurence.Johanson@uksh.de

Introduction: Interactions between G protein-coupled receptors (GPCR) and their endogenous ligands orchestrate a myriad of cellular events, among them cell trafficking and migration. Further, altered expression of GPCR and their ligands has been implicated in different autoimmune and inflammatory diseases. Apart from natural ligands, it has recently been shown that autoantibodies targeting GPCR might play a role in inflammatory and autoimmune diseases such as systemic sclerosis (SSc). Based upon previous findings it is assumed that high concentrations of anti-CXCR3 and anti-CXCR4 antibodies act in a protective manner, while high concentrations of anti-ETAR and anti-AT1R aggravate inflammatory mechanisms. We want to show those effect of antibodies against CXCR3, CXCR4, ETAR and AT1R in a murine model of atherosclerosis.

Methods: We injected IgG preparations containing different levels of autoantibodies directed against CXCR3/4 or ETAR and AT1R from patients with SSc and from healthy controls into a passive murine model of atherosclerosis (C57BL/6, Apoe-/-, high fat diet). Using red oil staining of the atherosclerotic plaques in the aorta, flow cytometry, differential blood count via Vet abc plus, ELISA and immunohistology analyses, it will be examined if those IgG preparations are able to modify leukocyte migration into different tissues like lung and spleen in comparison to peripheral blood.

DOI: 10.18416/RAB.2018.1809029   Advances in RAB Research • Article ID: 1809029

Results: Preliminary findings of the ELISA indicates migration of leukocytes into the spleen modulated by the anti-GPCR IgG. More preliminary findings, like some results of the red oil staining and the flow cytometry analyses will be shown.

Conclusion: We assume an interplay between anti-AT1R/anti-ETAR & anti-CXCR3/4 and their receptors mediates organotropism of leukocytes in inflammatory & autoimmune diseases. In addition, membrane extracts of CHO cells overexpressing CXCR3/4, ETAR and AT1R will be applied in the same murine model to compare passive and active immunization schemes.

DOI: 10.18416/RAB.2018.1809029   Advances in RAB Research • Article ID: 1809029

Autoantibodies targeting muscarinic acetylcholine receptors: implications on fatigue in systemic sclerosis

Sabine Sommerlatte[a,*], Hannah Bittern[a], Silke Pitann[a], Gabriele Marschner[a], Antje Müller[a], Otavio Cabral-Marques[a], Harald Heidecke[b], Tanja Lange[a], Gabriela Riemekasten[a]

[a] Department of Rheumatology and clinical Immunology, University Medical Center Schleswig-Holstein, Lübeck, Germany
[b] CellTrend GmbH Luckenwalde, Germany
* Corresponding author, email: sabine.sommerlatte@uksh.de

Introduction: Muscarinic acetylcholine receptors (mAChR) are neuroimmune G protein-coupled receptors comprising 5 subtypes (M1-M5). Autoantibodies recognizing mAChRs have been linked to chronic fatigue syndrome. Fatigue is common in patients with autoimmune diseases such as systemic sclerosis (SSc) and is frequently ranked as one of the most wearing symptoms.

Methods: In a first study, we analyzed autoantibodies targeting M1-M5 in 113 SSc patients and 113 gender- and age-matched healthy controls by ELISA. In an ongoing second study we apply self-report questionnaires to investigate frequency and severity of fatigue (brief fatigue inventory, multidimensional fatigue inventory 20, fatigue severity scale), depression (patient health questionnaire-9), pain (numeric rating scales), sleepiness (epworth sleepiness scale), sleep quality (pittsburgh sleep quality index) and chronotype (munich chronotype questionnaire) in relation to anti-M1-M5 autoantibodies in 100 SSc patients.

Results: In the first study we found significantly decreased levels of autoantibodies targeting M2, M4 and M5 in SSc patients compared to healthy controls. In the second study, 72 SSc patients have completed the questionnaires until now. 24% of these patients suffered from severe fatigue and 49% felt unusually fatigued during the last week. 33% showed at least mild depression, 59% enhanced sleepiness and 63% poor sleep quality. Fatigue correlated significantly with depression, sleepiness and pain. Data on chronotype and autoantibodies are currently under analysis.

Conclusion: Our findings demonstrate a high frequency of fatigue, depression, sleepiness and poor sleep in SSc patients. Altered patterns of autoantibodies targeting mAChR may contribute to the pathogenesis of fatigue in SSc and potentially offer new therapeutic possibilities.

Role of anti-alpha-adrenoceptor autoantibodies and leukocytic alpha-adrenoceptors in primary Raynaud's phenomenon

Catharina Frahm[a,*], Anja Kerstein[a], Silke Pitann[a], Sara Comdühr[a], Harald Heidecke[b], Antje Müller[a], Tanja Lange[a], Gabriela Riemekasten[a]

[a] *Department of Rheumatology and clinical Immunology, University Medical Center Schleswig-Holstein, Germany*
[b] *CellTrend GmbH, Luckenwalde, Germany*
[*] *Corresponding author, email: Catharina.Frahm@uksh.de*

Introduction: α2C-adrenoceptors expressed by vascular smooth muscle cells recognize circulating norepinephrine and in this way contribute to local and systemic cold-induced vasoconstriction. Primary Raynaud's phenomenon (pRP) is being considered as exaggerated cold-induced vasoconstriction. We hypothesize that autoantibodies targeting vascular and leukocytic α-adrenoceptor subtypes may represent a mechanism leading to pRP.

Methods: Peripheral blood and serum were obtained from patients with pRP (n=20) and age- and sexmatched healthy controls (HC, n=10). pRP was diagnosed using nailfold capillaroscopy and a questionnaire based upon published International Consensus Criteria. Circulating anti-α1/α2-adrenoceptor autoantibodies were measured by ELISA. Peripheral blood mononuclear cells (PBMC) and neutrophils (PMN) were isolated using Ficoll gradient and MACS-based separation technique, respectively. α2A, 2B, 2C-adrenoceptor mRNA and protein expressions were analyzed by qPCR and Western blot.

Results: Both, circulating anti-α1- and anti-α2-adrenoceptor autoantibodies were present in HC and patients with pRP. While the concentration of anti-α1- was higher than that of anti-α2-antibodies in HC, there were no differences between HC and pRP regarding the concentrations of anti-?1 and anti-α2-antibodies. However, clinical characteristics of pRP correlate with anti-α2-antibodies. PMN and PBMC of both, HC and patients with pRP expressed mRNA for α2A-, α2B- and α2C-adrenoceptors. In terms of protein expression, a different expression of α2A, α2B and α2C-adrenoceptor was observed in PMN and PBMC of pRP when compared to HC.

Conclusion: It is assumed that autoantibodies recognizing α-adrenoceptor subtypes act as ligands on these receptors and modulate the vasoconstriction of small vessels, especially in the fingers of patients with pRP leading to vasospastic episodes.

DOI: 10.18416/RAB.2018.1809031   Advances in RAB Research • Article ID: 1809031

Inflamed tissue contributes to the emergence of auto-reactivity in granulomatosis with polyangiitis

Gesche Weppner[a,*], Olena Ohlei[b], Christoph M. Hammers[c], Konstanze Holl-Ulrich[d],
Jan Voswinkel[e], Julia Bischof, Katrin Hasselbacher[f], Gabriela Riemekasten[a],
Peter Lamprecht[a], Saleh Ibrahim[c], Christof Iking-Konert[g], Andreas Recke[c], Antje Müller[c]

[a] Department of Rheumatology & Clinical Immunology, Lübeck, Germany
[b] Lübeck Interdisciplinary platform for Genome Analytics - Institute of Neurogenetics, Lübeck, Germany
[c] Department of Dermatology, Lübeck, Germany
[d] Institute of Pathology - Marienkrankenhaus, Hamburg, Germany
[e] Medical Faculty - University of Saarland, Saarbrücken, Germany
[f] Department of Otorhinolaryngology, Lübeck, Germany
[g] Dpt. of Rheumatology & Immunology, Bad Bramstedt, Germany
* Corresponding author, email: Gesche.Weppner@uksh.de

Introduction: Circulating anti-neutrophilic cytoplasmic autoantibodies targeting proteinase 3 (PR3-ANCA) are a diagnostic and pathogenic hallmark of granulomatosis with polyangiitis (GPA). It is, however, incompletely understood if inflamed tissue supports presence and emergence of PR3-ANCA+ B-cells.

Methods: In search of such cells in inflamed tissue of GPA, immunofluorescence staining for IgG and a common PR3-ANCA idiotype (5/7 Id) was undertaken. To gain insight into surrogate markers possibly indicative of a PR3-driven antibody response at inflamed sites, a meta-analysis comprising IGVH and IGVL genes derived from respiratory tract tissue of GPA (231 clones) was performed. Next generation sequencing-based IGHV genes derived from peripheral blood of healthy donors (244.353 clones) and previously published IGLV genes (148 clones) served as controls. For comparison, Ig genes of murine and known human monoclonal anti-PR3 antibodies were analyzed.

Results: Few 5/7 Id+ / IgG+ B-cells were detected in inflamed tissue of GPA. IGHV and IGLV genes derived from inflamed tissue of GPA displayed altered V(D)J usage, contributing to prolonged complementarity determining region 3 (CDR3) in the IGHV genes. Further, selection against amino acid exchanges was prominent in the framework region of IGHV genes derived from inflamed tissue of GPA. Comparing V(D)J rearrangements and deduced amino acid sequences of the CDR3 between anti-PR3 antibodies and Ig clones derived from inflamed tissue of GPA, yielded no identities and few similarities. Thus, few PR3-ANCA+ B-cells were found in inflamed tissue of GPA.

Conclusion: Notably, the search for clones producing PR3-ANCA IgG in inflamed tissue might require methods that can detect rare clones.

DOI: 10.18416/RAB.2018.1809032   Advances in RAB Research • Article ID: 1809032

New insights into the diagnostics of autoantibodies against G-protein coupled receptors – pitfalls in the autoantibody detection

Annekathrin Haberland[a,*], Johannes Müller[a], Gerd Wallukat[a], Katrin Wenzel[a]

[a] Berlin Cures GmbH
* Corresponding author, email: haberland@berlincures.de

Introduction: The knowledge about the impact of functionally acting autoantibodies which target G-protein coupled receptors (GPCR-AABs) is steadily growing. GPCR-AABs activate receptors; physiological counter-regulation, as known from natural ligands, does, however, not occur. This leads to pathological consequences such as heart failure (here AABs against the beta1-adrenoceptor, beta1-AABs) or other diseases. The problem with the detection of these GPCR-AABs is A) their low titers and B) their functional activity. A) For autoantibodies against the TSH-receptor (Grave's disease) a bioassay (cAMP cascade) revealed titers between 0.0005 and 0.006% of the IgG fraction [Nakatake et al., Thyroid. 2006;16: 1077]. For most of the other GPCR-AABs almost nothing is known about the titer. B) With respect to the functional activity, binding without receptor activation has already been described [Bornholz et al., Cardiovasc Res. 2013;97: 472]. We here tested, if such factors influence on the GPCR-AAB detection.

Methods: A bioassay [Wenzel et al., Heliyon. 2017;3: e00362] and a previously published ELISA [Nagatomo et al., J Am Coll Cardiol. 2017;69: 968] for the detection of the functional activity and the binding of beta1-AABs, respectively, were exploited.

Results: Using the bioassay, beta1-AAB samples were identified and assigned to their epitopes on the receptor using mapping peptides. The samples were also applied onto an ELISA which was specifically developed and previously exploited for a large study investigating "Myocardial Recovery in Patients With Systolic Heart Failure and Autoantibodies Against β1-Adrenergic Receptors" [Nagatomo et al.]. The comparison revealed that the ELISA results did not match the bioassay outcome.

Conclusion: Since the existence of GPCR-AABs is increasingly gaining clinical importance and plays a decisive role in therapeutic decisions, erroneous measurements can have an enormous impact on patient therapy decisions. That is the reason why reliable tests have to be established which are able to identify the functional active GPCR AABs.

Infinite Science
Publishing

Network-based analysis reveals signatures of IgG autoantibodies targeting G protein-coupled receptors in health and disease

P08

Otavio Cabral-Marques[a], Alexandre Marques[a], Lasse Melvær Giil[b], Roberta de Vito[c],
Barbara Elizabeth Engelhardt[c], Jalid Sehouli[d], Harald Heidecke[e], Gabriela Riemekasten[a,*]

DOI: 10.18416/RAB.2018.1809002   Advances in RAB Research • Article ID: 1809002

β1-adrenergic receptor autoantibody levels are higher in patients with Graves' hyperthyroidism than in matched healthy controls and decrease after anti-thyroid treatment

P09

Anna Lundgren[a,*], Karin Tammelin[b], Mats Holmberg[c], Helena Filipsson Nyström[d]

DOI: 10.18416/RAB.2018.1809005   Advances in RAB Research • Article ID: 1809005

Patterns of 31 new autoantibodies against G-protein-coupled receptors and growth factors

P10

H. Bittern[a], A. Carvalho-Marques[a], C. Fouodo[a], I. König[a], S. Schinke[a,*], O. Cabral-Marques[a],
H. Heidecke[b], G. Riemekasten[a]

DOI: 10.18416/RAB.2018.1809006   Advances in RAB Research • Article ID: 1809006

Transfer of PBMC from SSc patients to immunodeficient mice leads to the production of autoantibodies against AT1R and ETAR

P11

Xiaoyang Yue[a], Yaqing Shu[a], Junie Tchudjin Magatsin[a], Xiaoqing Wang[a], Junping Yin Marjan Ahmadi[a], Harald Heidecke[b], Brigitte Kasper[a], Xinhua Yu[a], Frank Petersen[a,*], Gabriela Riemekasten[*]

DOI: 10.18416/RAB.2018.1809011   Advances in RAB Research • Article ID: 1809011

Sialylated autoantigen-reactive IgG antibodies attenuate disease development in mouse models of lupus nephritis and rheumatoid arthritis

P12

Yannic C. Bartsch, Johann Rahmöller, Alexei Leliavski, Gina-Maria Lilienthal, Janina Petry, Marc Ehlers[*]

DOI: 10.18416/RAB.2018.1809015   Advances in RAB Research • Article ID: 1809015

Autoantibodies targeting complement receptors 3a and 5a are decreased in ANCA-associated vasculitis

P13

Sebastian Klapa[a,*], Andreas Koch[b], Anja Kerstein[a], Christian Karsten[c], Harald Heidecke[d], Markus Huber-Lang[e], Peter Lamprecht[a], Gabriela Riemekasten[a], Antje Müller[a]

DOI: 10.18416/RAB.2018.1809016   Advances in RAB Research • Article ID: 1809016

Impact of regulatory (auto-)antibodies against G-protein-coupled receptors on blood pressure in women ten years after early-onset preeclampsia

P14

Anna Birukov[a,d,e,f,g,*], Hella Muijsers[c], Harald Heidecke[b], Nadine Haase[a,d,e,f,g], Kristin Kräker[a,d,e,f,g], Dominik N. Müller[a,d,e,f,g], Florian Herse[a,d,e,f,g], Angela Maas[c], Ralf Dechend[a,d,e,f,g,h]

DOI: 10.18416/RAB.2018.1809017   Advances in RAB Research • Article ID: 1809017

Autoantibodies in serum of systemic scleroderma patients: peptide-based epitope mapping indicates increased binding to cytoplasmic domains of CXCR3

P15

Andreas Recke[a], Ann-Katrin Regensburger[b,*], Florian Weigold[c], Antje Müller[d], Harald Heidecke[e], Gabriele Marschner[d], Christoph M. Hammers[a], Ralf J. Ludwig[b], Gabriela Riemekasten[b]

DOI: 10.18416/RAB.2018.1809025   Advances in RAB Research • Article ID: 1809025

Detection and functional characterization of angiotensin receptor Type 1 autoantibodies: establishment and clinical translation

P16

Valérie Boivin-Jahns[a,*], Chistina Zechmeister[a], Claudia Schuetz[a], Martin J. Lohse[b], Roland Jahns[c], Xinhua Yu[d], Frank Petersen[d], Stefanie Hahner[e], Martin Fassnacht[e]

DOI: 10.18416/RAB.2018.1809026   Advances in RAB Research • Article ID: 1809026

Disclosure of cooperation

Disclosure of payments made during the 2nd RAB-Symposium

In accordance with transparency obligations, we transparently present the services and the extent of support provided by companies to participants both in announcing and holding the congress.

Institution	Sponsoring	Service
Euroimmun AG	5.000 €	Industrial exhibition, Marketing
CellTrend GmbH	3.000 €	Industrial exhibition, Marketing
MSD SHARP & DOHME GMBH	2.000 €	Industrial exhibition, Marketing
Bristol-Myers Squibb GmbH & Co. KGaA	2.000 €	Industrial exhibition, Marketing
Celgene GmbH	2.000 €	Industrial exhibition, Marketing
Sanofi-Aventis Deutschland GmbH	2.000 €	Industrial exhibition, Marketing
Actelion Pharmaceuticals Deutschland GmbH	1.500 €	Industrial exhibition, Marketing
Novartis Pharma GmbH	1.400 €	Industrial exhibition, Marketing
Miltenyi Biotec GmbH	1.000 €	Industrial exhibition, Marketing
Lilly Deutschland GmbH	1.000 €	Industrial exhibition, Marketing
Chugai Pharma Europe Ltd.	1.000 €	Industrial exhibition, Marketing
Roche Pharma GmbH	1.000 €	Industrial exhibition, Marketing
GlaxoSmithKline GmbH & Co. KG	1.000 €	Industrial exhibition, Marketing
Janssen-Cilag GmbH	1.000 €	Industrial exhibition, Marketing
Hexal AG	1.000 €	Industrial exhibition, Marketing
Shire Baxalta Deutschland GmbH	750 €	Industrial exhibition, Marketing
AbbVie Deutschland GmbH & Co. KG	500 €	Marketing

Infinite Science | Publishing

www.ingramcontent.com/pod-product-compliance
Lightning Source LLC
Chambersburg PA
CBHW081547220326
41598CB00036B/6589